Overcoming Common Problems Series

The Chronic Pain Diet Book

NEVILLE SHONE

sheldon PRESS

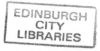

First published in Great Britain in 2008

Sheldon Press
36 Causton Street
London SW1P 4ST

The author and publisher have made every effort to ensure
that the external website and email addresses included in this book are
correct and up to date at the time of going to press. The author
and publisher are not responsible for the contents, quality or
continuing accessibility of the sites.

British Library Cataloguing-in-Publication Data
A catalogue record for this book is available from the British Library

ISBN 978-1-84709-024-9

1 3 5 7 9 10 8 6 4 2

Typeset by Pantek Arts Ltd, Maidstone, Kent
Printed in Great Britain by Ashford Colour Press

Contents

About the author

Neville Shone was at the height of his career as a university teacher and researcher, bringing up a young family, a keen sportsman and amateur entertainer, when an operation to remove a spinal tumour rendered him almost immobile and in constant pain. His career and social life ended abruptly, bringing him close to despair. This is reflected in his book *Coping Successfully with Pain*, first published by Sheldon Press in 1992, but the real story is about his fight back and the techniques of pain management which enabled him to regain his mobility, his zest for life, and to escape from his prison of pain. After several revisions, *Coping Successfully with Pain* is now in its third edition, in which Neville Shone included a chapter on the relationship between diet and chronic pain. *The Chronic Pain Diet Book* continues this theme and is based on the 15 years' research he has made into the subject. Neville continues to help people caught up in the pain trap through his involvement with pain charities. He has appeared on many radio and television programmes on the subject of pain and has acted as adviser to a number of TV documentary makers. Neville is also the author of *Cancer – a Family Affair*, published by Sheldon Press in 1995.

Foreword

I have known Neville for almost 15 years and it was very early into our working friendship that we discussed the development of pain management programmes for delivery in the community. With his personal experience of chronic pain and his involvement in the development of the chronic pain services at Walton Hospital, Liverpool, it was a natural progression for him to write a manual for the Pain Association that became the basis of the first community based pain management programme in the UK.

The Pain Association Scotland has gone on to develop this programme through a network of 34 self management groups in Scotland and 3 in Northumberland. Our staff led courses are designed for people with any form of chronic pain, irrespective of diagnosis. The focus of the programme is to build self management skills leading to a reduction in pain, positive change, and an improved quality of life and wellbeing. This has an impact not only on the group members but also on the carers and families.

I remember all these years ago discussing diet and in particular at that time coffee. Owing to the stress of my previous employment I had become extremely reliant upon caffeine. Already into the research of products, Neville explained that with coffee it was not just the caffeine that was the problem but the acid content in the coffee. Discussions with Neville over the years have given me an insight into the problems that many products have upon us all.

Just over two years ago my first grandchild was born and was failing to thrive. It became obvious that she was intolerant of dairy products. Unfortunately, she became extremely ill before the 'powers that be' would acknowledge this. However, a change onto a protein free baby formula solved the problem and she is now being a happy, thriving two year old.

Generally, the foods we crave, particularly when we are inactive and feeling low, are the ones that are going to have the most negative impact on health. If left unrecognised they continue to fuel the pain, depression, anxiety and isolation.

The contents of this book are well researched and, more importantly they are based on a very personal journey to which I am sure many readers will relate, as in the case of Neville's first book

Coping Successfully with Pain.
Although the concept of food sensitivity is not a new one, few people will recognise that it can have such an impact on their pain. The information on the effects of food types and suggested diet changes, while not promising a cure, carry the possibility of an improvement in quality of life and enable many readers to cope better with their chronic pain condition.

David Falconer
Director
Pain Association Scotland

Acknowledgements

I wish to express my thanks to David Falconer, Director, Pain Association Scotland, for agreeing to write the Foreword. In my capacity as patron of Pain Association Scotland I have worked with David for many years and I have been encouraged by his enthusiasm and tenacity in ensuring that the organization, through its groups in the community, works towards achieving the goal of establishing the best possible service for people with chronic pain.

I also wish to express my thanks to the following people throughout Europe who have helped me with translations:

- Eliana of Infusions Restaurant, Kendal, Cumbria, who also went out of her way to prepare delicious food suited to my diet.
- Gloria Moro and husband Valeriano – also for their hospitality and for showing us the delights of Spanish food and culture.
- Flora Morhmann – also for her friendship and hospitality over the past 15 years, and for the book *The Real Food of China*, which we use a lot.
- Patricia Bonet-Hancox of Bonterra Park – also for her kindness and concern for our well-being.
- Erna Bruwier – also for her friendship; and Jürgen (Jo) Riechers – also for friendship and for making sure everything was 'vertical'.
- Paulo Torres of Laithwaites, part of Direct Wines Ltd, for going out of his way to assist me with information about additives even though he knew I was critical of the practice.

I also wish to express my thanks to the following people:

- Joanna Moriarty and Fiona Marshall of Sheldon Press who have encouraged me in my writing and given me the opportunity to reach a largely forgotten group in the community.
- Mr R. J. Mewis, chiropractor, who in the last few months has used his skills to repair damage following a fall. His work enabled me to sit comfortably and carry on with the book.
- My wife Eve, who insisted that I stop talking about writing this book and get down to work. She has not only worked on the recipes and helped with the research over the past 15 years, but has typed this book at least three times when it has undergone several revisions as a result of second and third thoughts. Without her help this book would not have been written.

Author's note

None of my work is subsidized and it is completely independent of any commercial assistance or reward. I accept full responsibility for the views expressed. Readers are encouraged at all times to seek medical advice for their condition and, above all, not to give up any medication without consultation with their doctors.

Introduction

Chronic pain affects more than 8.5 million people in the UK. It costs the economy £18 billion a year in lost working days. An estimated 30 per cent of the population – up to 70 million per cent – also suffer in the USA, where it is said to be the most costly health problem. Yet, according to one study, two out of three per cent with chronic pain say that their medication is not adequate and 96 per cent of general practitioners believe there is significant room for improvement in treatment. Another survey found that between one-half and two-thirds of people with chronic pain are less able or unable to exercise, enjoy normal sleep, perform household chores, attend social activities, drive a car or walk. One-quarter of them experience broken or strained relationships with family and friends. When you consider that we have an ageing population, these figures become alarming. As you might expect, the numbers of people with chronic pain increase with age and almost 25 per cent of those aged over 65 suffer from this type of pain. It seems rather sad that, at a time when people are living so much longer, the only thing they can look forward to is a life limited by pain and suffering. Neck pain, back pain, arthritis, allergies and depression are listed as the top five chronic health problems.

This book results from 15 years' experience and research into the link between food sensitivities and chronic pain. It looks at how eating certain foods may result in inflammation, water retention and swelling, fatigue, muscle weakness, and being overweight and can aggravate chronic pain. It suggests a combination of foods that not only reduce the pain but lead to an unparalleled level of health and activity.

In my book *Coping Successfully with Pain* I highlighted my own experience of breaking out of the prison of pain, depression, immobility and isolation, and I attempted to guide the reader to discover ways of coming to terms with chronic pain – to cope with the emotional and social consequences and to make lifestyle changes, building on a programme of exercise and relaxation that makes it possible to lead a full and active life. In the third edition of that book there is a chapter on the relationship between food and pain. This new book carries on where that left off.

This is a highly personalized account showing how difficult it can be to lead a full and active life when one is coping not only with pain but with many food sensitivities that, in their turn, aggravate the pain, causing inflammation, retention of water, swelling, fatigue and muscle weakness – which at one time caused me to revert to immobility and to the need to use a wheelchair. It took a long time to understand the process because initially all the difficulties were thought to be associated with the original chronic pain problem. Drugs were out of the question because of my intolerance to the usual pain-killers and anti-inflammatory agents. The chance reading of a book in Canada led my wife and me to investigate the possible involvement of food in the problem. Eventually, with help, we were able to identify the foods that were more likely to trigger the symptoms and eventually we arrived at a combination of foods that not only reduced the pain but also led to a level of health and activity that I had not experienced in 30 years.

The concept of food sensitivity is important. Many illnesses, in particular arthritis, multiple sclerosis (MS), migraine and other conditions characterized by inflammation, are thought to be closely related to food sensitivity. It is possible to go on for many years, perhaps almost a lifetime, unaware that even your favourite food or drink can cause such unpleasant problems. No symptoms may occur until some stressful event or period in your life poses a severe challenge. This is an important subject that I shall develop at some length because it is my belief that chronic illness and pain, stress and the food we eat are inextricably linked, and unless this is understood and changes are made, the person with chronic pain or illness can be precipitated into a downward spiral and give up altogether.

Food is an emotional subject and often has deep meaning to families, particularly where a mother expresses her love of the family through the meals she so lovingly prepares. The society we live in plays a big part in determining what we eat, how it is prepared, and how and when we eat it. These things make it difficult to cope with food sensitivity and to make the changes necessary to re-establish health.

Using my own life experience I shall stress the importance of parents listening to their children and observing their reactions to the food they are offered and I shall attempt to guide readers to listen to their body as a way of recognizing their individual problems. It is so easy to ignore signs of what appear to be minor internal discomforts when you are coping with a major chronic pain problem. It is so easy to get indigestion and pop in an antacid tablet or to have chronic constipation and take a laxative and then carry on – until the next time! So advice will be given on recognizing early symptoms.

In the following pages I attempt to show how foods can be used to heal, to change the pain state and to prevent problems and illness from developing. As I have had to cope with pain and the discomforts of food sensitivities I want to share my experience and make suggestions for simple first-aid measures to deal with adverse reactions to food without recourse to drugs.

Over the years Eve and I have worked together on finding a diet that suits us both. It might not suit everybody because I do believe that everyone needs to be encouraged to discover foods that give maximum possible nutrition. No two people are the same and that goes for our nutritional needs. Most of us soldier on, eating what is put on the family table and conforming to the diet prescribed by our family or culture. It does not follow that if we do this we are going to gain full nutritional benefits.

The recipes presented are designed to provide a base on which you can build your own diet. People with chronic illness who are faced with cutting out certain foods have to ensure that they suffer no deficiencies in nutrition. The recipes take this into account. Eve and I are sure that you will find the suggestions not only nutritious but attractive and, above all, tasty. Knowing that people with chronic pain are likely to have low energy levels and physical limitations, the ingredients are kept simple and easily sourced and do not take long to prepare.

If you do have the courage to make changes to your diet, I am confident that you will surprise yourself and move on to a new level of health and fitness. I am not in any way promising that you will be 'cured' of your problems, in the same way that I make no claim that I have found a 'cure'. My medical condition still remains and I must work hard to maintain a good level of fitness, but the difference I notice is that many of the more frightening features of my problems have disappeared and I have developed a confidence that has enabled me to move away from an isolated, withdrawn position. I am convinced that working on food sensitivities and making sure that I do not eat the wrong food for me has brought about this change. There can be no other explanation. If you are setting out to control your pain and seek improvements, I have no doubt that you will be able to make use of the guidance on shopping and eating out in restaurants at home and abroad because, like me, you are likely to feel you want to spread your wings and get back into enjoying normal social activities.

1

Oh dear! What can the matter be? . . .

Shortly after completing the book *Coping Successfully with Pain* I found I was losing much of my hard-won mobility in spite of maintaining a daily schedule of exercise and relaxation. I was finding it impossible to drive for more than 10 minutes before I was overwhelmed by pain and fatigue. As a passenger I was asking my wife to stop driving every 30 minutes so that I could move around to ease the pain. I recorded in 1994 that I had severe pain when putting my feet to the ground and that when out and about I found myself staggering, with no control over my legs. All the strength had gone out of them. As well as being painful it was most embarrassing because the self-help methods that I cherished and followed almost slavishly appeared not to be working.

I was so weak I could not climb the stairs to bed and had to sleep downstairs. Most nights I woke with profuse sweating and would often go into a hypothermic state. From time to time I had what might be called asthma attacks although I had never been an asthma sufferer, and I had extremely painful muscle spasms that severely restricted my movement. I had no idea what the problem might be. My medical advisers told me that these symptoms were what might be expected given my history of pain resulting from spinal stenosis, arthritis and, in particular, nerve damage and scar tissue from a spinal operation some years earlier for the removal of a benign tumour. My pain and arthritis could not be treated by any of the pain-killers or anti-inflammatory drugs, most of which are based on aspirin.

Since my teens I had suffered digestive discomfort including stomach bleeding in the days before it was recognized that some people are allergic to aspirin. I was put on a milk diet and advised to take antacids for the rest of my life.

One medical practitioner actually voiced her opinion: 'You have not got much going for you, have you?' After I got over my anger at such a tactless comment, I began to think about the periods in my life when I felt really well and found it difficult to pinpoint such a time. I remembered that periods of fitness and high energy were very soon interrupted by longer periods of feeling 'one degree under' accompanied by back and leg pains and migraines. Sometimes, when working or enjoying my hobbies, I would get the feeling that things that I had been doing effortlessly were now draining my energy. In spite of this I had performed well in school and at university; I had been an athlete and enjoyed the outdoor life as well as singing and acting and had progressed in my profession.

2

Was it something I ate?

Reflecting on my health history, I asked my general practitioner whether my problems had anything to do with my food in view of the fact that diet was considered to be very important in controlling the inflammation and pain of stomach ulcers. 'Of course not!' was the emphatic reply. 'Just keep eating a healthy balanced diet.' At that time I did not question the doctor but on my way home I thought, 'What is a healthy diet? What is a balanced diet?' To me this meant a fair intake of protein – meat, milk, cheese, eggs and fish; carbohydrates – bread, potatoes, cereals; vegetables and fibre; and fats – butter or margarine (which was then being advocated as being healthier than butter). At that time I was getting all of these things and could not see any problems with my diet.

It was while coming to terms with these issues and an ever-increasing loss of mobility that we decided to keep our promise to visit elderly relatives in Canada whom we had not seen for many years. While visiting a bookshop in Toronto I discovered the *Dairy-Free Cookbook* by Jane Zukin (published by Prima Publishing of California). I do not know why I chose to open this book and browse through it other than idle curiosity, but as I turned the pages I read about milk allergy and lactose intolerance and how they showed themselves from infancy onwards.

I instantly recognized myself and some of my problems and decided there and then to cut out all dairy products from my diet to see whether this made a difference. Within just a matter of days I could feel the difference: no more wheeziness, no more stomach discomfort, an increase in energy and the beginnings of an improvement in mobility.

Although my pain levels did not improve dramatically, I had less stiffness in my joints, particularly my hands, and was aware that I was experiencing more good days than I had previously. While I was having dairy products I always awoke sore and stiff and it took almost two hours for this pain and stiffness to wear off. Showering and dressing always left me exhausted. Within a week or two of cutting out dairy products my mornings improved and dressing and showering were not such an ordeal.

However, some of my problems remained and I tended to treat these as 'set-backs' in my general progress. (Those of you who have read *Coping Successfully with Pain* will know that there is a chapter dealing with 'set-backs' and how to cope with them.) I could go for days without experiencing any difficulties and at first assumed the work I was doing on my 'set-backs' was working. What worried me was that each repetition of my symptoms was becoming progressively more severe. I began to get suspicious that there were other reasons for my all-too-frequent 'set-backs' and that apart from dairy products there might be other foods to which I was sensitive.

From this point I began to experiment with my diet and to read widely on the subject of nutrition in order to explore the possibility that there was a relationship between diet and chronic pain.

When I first started my research my sole intention was to follow up my own suspicions that my pain problem was connected with the food I ate. My research and the consequent changes that I have made in my diet have resulted in a real improvement in my pain condition and, as a bonus, an improvement in my general health and outlook on life. As I got deeper into the subject I realized that the connection between diet and pain was so vital and so complex that I should continue my work in order to produce a book for the benefit of other pain sufferers.

3

Chronic pain defined

It is important to understand what is meant by 'chronic pain'. Chronic pain can be defined as pain that is persistent and constant rather than intermittent. It may be severe at times but at other times it may be dull and at a level that is enough to remind you of its presence, gnawing away at your stamina and reducing your drive and initiative. It has been recognized as an illness in itself by the medical profession and the Department of Health since the early 1990s. Like any other chronic illness, it is long-standing, lasting for months or years rather than days or weeks. The term 'chronic pain' is used by the medical profession when pain has been present for more than six months.

Problems that give rise to short bursts of pain, perhaps on a weekly or monthly basis, include such things as migraine, tension headaches, forms of neuralgia and premenstrual pain. Quite often such pain can be extremely severe and debilitating even though it might last only for a few hours or days. This kind of pain may be referred to as 'chronic periodic pain'. Although it might be possible to carry on normally for most of the time, it can begin to dominate the way the person lives, feels, thinks and behaves, reducing the capacity to enjoy life – in just the same way as chronic pain does.

It is generally accepted that initially pain is a signal that the body is under attack, a normal response to cuts and bruises, broken bones, knocks and internal injury. It can be a sign of a disease process, or it can follow surgery or it can be an alarm that calls for attention. If the cause of the pain is treated appropriately it goes away. Pain of this nature is short-lived, lasting no longer than six months at the outside, and is usually referred to as acute pain; it is regarded as 'useful' pain. This is in contrast to the pain that arrives too late to warn us – for example, cancer pain, which may come long after the disease process is established and as such may be regarded as 'useless' pain. Chronic pain that continues, sometimes in the absence of illness or injury or long after healing has taken place, may also be regarded as 'useless' pain but, of course, this type of pain also needs attention and should not be dismissed.

Conditions giving rise to chronic pain include:

- rheumatoid arthritis and osteoarthritis;
- osteoporosis;
- spondylitis and spondylosis;
- spinal stenosis;
- fibromyalgia;
- myalgic encephalopathy (ME), also known as chronic fatigue syndrome;
- sciatica;
- facet joint pain;
- ruptured or bulging cervical discs causing severe back, head and neck pain, which can radiate down the arms and legs;
- tumours – malignant or non-malignant, which can cause nerve irritation;
- multiple sclerosis (MS);
- neuralgia – for example trigeminal neuralgia causing severe face pain, post-herpetic neuralgia (pain after shingles), post-operative adhesions, and adhesions following injury;
- scar tissue and tissue damage, which can produce nerve irritation leading to prolonged persistent pain;
- cancer pain and pain following cancer treatment.

There are other pains that are not easily explained, and extensive tests and investigations may not always reveal a specific cause. People who have been told that no reasons can be put forward for their pain are often devastated, feeling that it is being implied that their pain is imagined. This is not so. The pain is real. It is just that the cause is not easily identifiable or that the current state of knowledge is limited. Challenge anybody who tries to dismiss your pain as something you must expect as you get older: it ain't necessarily so! Consult someone who knows something about the problem of chronic pain!

As an example, it is only recently that it has been possible to give a proper diagnosis of fibromyalgia. This previously unidentified illness was known for its painful symptoms but there was no way it could be diagnosed with any precision. Seeking help for generalized, non-specific pain and aches, lack of energy, skin tenderness, stomach cramps and constantly feeling unwell caused feelings of helplessness in doctors and despair in the sufferers.

Chronic pain can also arise from migraine, as well as following an injury long after healing has taken place, and phantom limb pain exists long after an amputation. Other causes include repeated unaccountable muscle spasms, low back pain, recurring headaches, and neck and shoulder pain. Then there is pain resulting from standing or sitting badly, and repetitive strain injury arising from working in such a way that exceptional strain is persistently applied to one part of the body. Such problems may take a long time to develop but unless they are recognized and corrected they can lead to chronic pain conditions. Candidates for this type of problem are people who have to sit in one position for long periods or have to repeat the same hand movements over and over again every working day. Hairdressing is an occupation that can lead to such problems. Drivers also often develop problems that lead to chronic pain.

Some people may put muscles under too much tension by using more effort than is necessary when carrying out everyday tasks. As a result muscle spasm may occur, causing soft tissue damage, and unless the cause is remedied the pain will persist. It is possible to measure the amount of tension in muscles while they are being used, and it may be necessary to teach ways of using muscles more efficiently. Unless help is given it is possible that pain arising from this cause will persist and soft tissue injury will develop.

If you have a chronic pain problem then no doubt you will have been given tablets or some or all of the following investigations and treatments: X-rays or scans, physiotherapy, manipulation, injections or even one or more operations. You may, or may not, have been referred to a pain clinic, but probably you have never been referred to a pain management course to learn the skills of self-management – very few people have the opportunity to attend such courses because they exist in only a small number of hospitals throughout the country. If you live in Scotland you are more likely to have the opportunity to attend such a course under the auspices of a hospital or Pain Association Scotland, which runs community-based courses in more than 30 centres throughout Scotland. A high percentage of those who attend one of these courses learn to manage their pain successfully, either without drugs and other medical intervention or with less powerful drugs than they have been using. Such courses teach techniques of relaxation, physical exercise programmes, methods of releasing muscle tension, distraction strategies and ways of making necessary lifestyle changes. Those who attend also learn how to pace themselves more effectively and to save energy for the pleasurable things of life. Much emphasis is placed on becoming more active, spending more time in the company of other people and setting new goals.

All of these things help in coping more effectively with pain and at the same time help people to lose their sense of isolation and the depression that goes with the chronic pain state. A full account of pain management is given in my book *Coping Successfully with Pain*.

This present book is an account of how I have used diet and nutrition to add to my own armoury of weapons in the daily fight against chronic pain, and I can now claim that I feel and look fitter than I have at any time in the past 30 years in spite of having the same medical condition. Each person has to find a way that suits him or her best – I hope that this account will give you more options in your quest for ways to cope successfully with your own pain. If you follow the dietary recommendations there is much to be gained because, for the first time, you will be getting at the root cause of your problems. The nutritional approach is to be commended along with pain management methods. By combining these approaches you are more likely to become totally responsible for your own treatment and progress. There is no way the nutritional approach can damage your body, which might happen if you rely solely on increasingly larger doses of medication or even more powerful pharmaceutical remedies. While anti-inflammatory drugs and pain-killers will dampen down the pain, they will bring about no cure, neither will they do anything to heal you physically or emotionally or to restore your ability to function fully with the maximum possible quality of life. This book, like the earlier one, aims to release you from the limitations imposed by chronic pain and to show how it is possible to lead a richer life, setting more and more ambitious goals for yourself.

4

Making an assessment of your own diet and health

Do you have pain?

You may wish to make your own assessment of the foods you eat and decide for yourself whether your diet has any bearing on your pain. Ask yourself the following questions.

1 Does meat such as lamb, beef or pork feature more than once a week in your diet?
2 Do you eat bacon more than once a week?
3 Do you eat sausages, black pudding or pies more than once a week?
4 Do you eat cooked meats (e.g. ham, tongue, roast pork, brawn, haslet, corned beef) more than once a week?
5 Do you eat deep-fried food more than once a week? This includes anything from the fish and chip shop, burgers and doughnuts.
6 Do you have a take-away more than once a week?
7 Do you have more than two cups a day of tea and coffee?
8 Do you have sugary, fizzy drinks more than twice a week? Remember each can of cola contains the equivalent of nine teaspoons of sugar.
9 Do you eat cakes, biscuits and pastries more than twice a week? And do you eat more than one at a time?
10 Do you eat processed foods (e.g. tinned or packet ready meals, crisps) more than twice a week?
11 Do you eat cheese more than once a week?
12 Do you drink milk every day, in addition to what goes into your tea or coffee?
13 Do you take any other dairy produce (ice-cream, yoghurts, milk-based desserts, cream, butter)?
14 Do you have sugary cereals or add extra sugar to your cereals more than twice a week?
15 Do you eat chocolates or sweets?

For every 'Yes' answer score 1 point.

If you score 5 points or under you may wish to explore whether you could make some adjustments to your diet, especially if you eat large helpings and – for instance – if you have cheese, bacon, red meat and fried foods as the major part of your diet, perhaps even to the exclusion of vegetables and fruit.

Any score over 5 points is an indication that you need to make serious dietary changes.

Now, another set of questions for you to think about.

1   Are you taking prescription drugs (e.g. pain-killers, anti-inflammatory agents, steroids)?
2   Are you overweight by more than 3 kg (7 lb)?
3   Do you retain water? Do you have swollen legs and ankles?
4   Have you got any digestive problems (e.g. indigestion, heartburn, constipation, bloating, wind, acid reflux, hiatus hernia, irritable bowel syndrome)?
5   Do you take medication for digestive problems, either from your doctor or your pharmacist?
6   Do you have trouble sleeping?
7   Do you often feel depressed or suffer from anxiety states?
8   Are you on medication for sleep problems, anxiety or depression?
9   Are you inactive for most of the day?
10 Do you avoid the company of others?

If you have answered yes to any of these questions and you have a score of 5 points or more on the first list of questions, then the signals are loud and clear. You must make changes. The first set of answers should have given you some indication about the nutritional value of your diet. High-fat and high-sugar foods and over-reliance on alcohol must be eliminated from your diet if you are to remain healthy. These foods particularly contribute to obesity, heart disease and diabetes, and according to the findings of researchers in USA, they also contribute to furred-up arteries, which are associated with many back pain problems.

You will note that I have not asked about cigarette smoking. I am assuming that you are well aware of the dangers of smoking for general health and in particular for anyone who has a chronic pain problem.

Possible changes to your diet

Whether you have pain or not, you will find you are healthier if you make some changes to your diet.

Size of helpings

Think first of all about the size of your helpings. Think of having two potatoes instead of five or six. In particular, have a higher proportion of vegetables than meat. Potatoes, particularly chips, do not count as vegetables in a healthy diet.

Meat

Cut down on the frequency with which you have meat or bacon: no more than one portion of each in a week. This will help to limit the fatty deposits of cholesterol that build up in your arteries and eventually block them, leading to heart attacks, strokes and maybe even severe back pain. If you cannot manage without meat in your diet then stick to rabbit or poultry, although modern production methods mean that chicken has a high proportion of fat, whereas once it was considered to be very lean. Wherever possible buy organic, free-range chicken.

Fish

It is suggested by the Department of Health that if you eat fish it should be one of the oily varieties (e.g. herring, mackerel, salmon). Their recommendation is that you should eat three portions a week, but they do not specify if this is in addition to or in place of any meat that you are eating now. I think it is wiser to think of fish as just another type of meat and, where possible, to eat oily fish in place of other meats because its omega-3 oil content makes it a much healthier alternative.

Dairy produce

Limit your intake of dairy produce – milk, cheese, yoghurt, milky puddings and cream. These too can add to the build-up of fatty deposits in the arteries. If you are milk- or lactose-intolerant then eliminate all dairy produce from your diet and substitute soya or rice milk products. Dairy products are known to contribute to the development of breast cancer, weight gain and possibly diabetes. They increase the amount of mucus, leading to sinus problems, lung congestion, wheeziness and snoring. By eliminating dairy produce and animal fats from your diet your chances of avoiding life-threatening illness are increased.

Evening snacks and meals

Limit the number of snacks you have in the evening. Try not to eat anything after 6.00 p.m. Cut out crisps because they contain so much salt and fat, and cut down on the number of pizzas and take-aways that you have. They are likely to be high in fat, especially if you order extra cheese, and they will certainly contain more salt than is good for you. A high salt intake can aggravate high blood pressure and lead to water retention, which, of course, will increase your weight. Just think that if you put on 3 kg (7 lb), it is equivalent to a bag of potatoes. Imagine the exhaustion of carrying around a bag of potatoes all day!

Bread

Limit the amount of bread you eat. Wheat flour is highly processed and is much stronger, with a higher gluten content, than it was 30 or 40 years ago. Gluten is a sticky substance contained in wheat that helps the flour to bind together and makes it easier to knead. The increased gluten is likely to irritate the bowel and can lead to wheat and gluten sensitivity and irritable bowel syndrome. Apart from this, too much bread will undoubtedly lead to weight gain. It is easy to control the amount of bread you eat. If you are accustomed to having sandwiches at lunchtime then make sure you do not eat toast at breakfast or teatime. Two rounds of bread a day are sufficient. When preparing this book I interviewed the baker in one of the better-known supermarkets. He confided that he would never eat the bread made in his bakery, nor would he give it to his children. He was concerned about the additives contained in the ready-made mixture that he had to work with. He made his own bread at home from ingredients over which he had complete control.

Processed foods

Naturally, it follows on from the above points that I suggest that you cut out or limit all processed foods. This includes cooked meats and factory-made frozen or dried meals. Much tinned food contains preservatives and colouring. Always look at the labels and choose tins that contain the least additives. For example, tinned peas need only contain peas, salt and water. Anything else is added to enhance the colour or the flavour, to give them a long shelf life or to disguise inferior quality of the basic ingredients. I have more to say about additives in Chapter 8.

Alcohol

Get control of the amount of alcohol you drink each day or each week. A glass of red wine is considered good for your heart in that it helps to break down cholesterol and improves blood flow, but two glasses do not produce twice the benefit! If you are a beer drinker, then you will know that too much produces unpleasant effects and quickly adds to your waist measurement! It is very difficult to lose this type of weight once it is there. Unfortunately, beer plays a major part in our culture, particularly when men gather together in groups: there seems to be some virtue in outdoing each other. Men are well known for 'mine is bigger than yours' competition. It certainly is true about the beer belly! Obesity, diabetes, high blood pressure and heart disease can start as a result of excessive drinking and, of course, any alcohol consumption will exacerbate a pain problem.

Sugars

Sugars include refined white sugar, icing sugar, caster sugar, raw cane sugar, glucose, sucrose, dextrose, maple syrup, honey, treacle and molasses. There is no difference nutritionally between these various kinds of sugar, which are commonly used on their own or as ingredients in cakes, biscuits, pastries, confectionery, cereals, bottled or canned drinks and cordials. They are used as sweeteners or to bring out the flavour of other ingredients in processed foods, even savoury ones. Sugars very quickly raise blood sugar levels, giving an uplift and an energy boost. This boost is short-lived and you can come down to earth very quickly, and you may feel the urge to take in more of the sugar-loaded food or drink. The body is unable to process large amounts of sugar and it is deposited in the cells, where it eventually turns into fat. Again, the result can be obesity, diabetes, heart disease or cancer. Fructose, on the other hand, is present in fruit and can be extracted to make a sweetener and does not produce the adverse effects of the other sugars mentioned above. It is always preferable to use fructose or even to prepare fruits to make a syrup that can be used as a sweetener for cakes and desserts. Some typical fructose-containing syrups are apple or pear concentrate, agave syrup (which comes from the same plant used to make tequila) and date syrup, which can be found in all good health-food shops. You can find in the recipe section (see p. 93) a way of making date purée, which can be used as a sweetener.

Fruit and vegetables

Most people can eat and benefit from all fruit and vegetables. They provide virtually all vitamins and minerals needed for good nutrition. The green vegetables in particular provide a full range of vitamins and minerals. The iron in plant products is absorbed much more easily when the body is low in iron. When the body has an ample supply, then iron from plant sources is not so readily absorbed. Meat contains a form of iron that cannot be regulated by the body and excess iron can be passed into the bloodstream even when the body has more than enough to cope with. As a result, iron from meat can increase the risk of heart problems whereas iron from plants never will. Make sure to include in your diet vegetables of all colours. The red and orange ones in particular contain bioflavinoids that help the body absorb and make use of vitamin C. Vegetables must become part of your daily diet, not just be used as a garnish. They should make up two-thirds of any meal that you have. The guidelines publicized in the UK recommend five portions of fruit or vegetables a day. From what I can gather from my research, a portion seems to relate to something the size of a medium-sized apple. In Australia the recommendation for daily consumption is almost double this level. You may find it difficult to imagine yourself eating so many vegetables or fruit in a day, but please remember that they are spread out over four or even five small meals. I find it helps to have some of my quota of fruit and vegetables in liquid form. There are various vegetable and pure fruit juices or smoothies on the market if you are unable to make your own. A word of caution! Do not buy fruit juice that contains sugar and always dilute pure fruit juice with 50 per cent water, since the juice on its own can be too strong for your system to cope with.

Grains

Foods made from grains – rice, oatmeal, barley, maize, wheat, quinoa, millet, bread and pasta – should provide a good base for your diet. In contrast to animal fats, whole grains are low in fat and high in fibre. They are a good source of protein and their carbohydrate content is released only slowly into the bloodstream rather than all at once, providing a source of energy and stamina that will last throughout the day. These low-fat foods improve the way in which insulin stops sugar building up in the blood. They do much to control the mechanisms that prevent diabetes. Anyone with food sensitivity to any of these grains will need to find a substitute.

Legumes

Legumes or pulses – the seed of pod-bearing plants (peas, beans, chickpeas, kidney beans and lentils) – are a good source of protein and fibre and are low in fat. The good news for pain sufferers is that they contain vitamin B6. It is known that in countries where people consume a lot of meat, poultry and fish, the diet is very high in animal protein, which uses up vitamin B6. A vegetable protein diet, on the other hand, supported by legumes and grains, allows the vitamin B6 to work. Vitamin B6 strengthens the nervous system so that it is more able to produce the chemicals that inhibit pain impulses. To enable the system to work in this way, it is necessary to reduce or even to exclude meat from the diet and to get most of your protein through grains and legumes. Do not expect instant pain relief. The benefits will probably be seen over a period of weeks.

Nuts and seeds

Nuts and seeds are very versatile in their use. They can be eaten raw or made into spreads and butters; chopped nuts and seeds can be used in virtually any recipe where a topping or crust is called for. They are high in protein, full of vitamins and minerals and the fat contained in them is rich in omega-3 oils. In particular, flaxseed oil has an anti-inflammatory effect and has a much greater omega-3 content than other nuts. Unlike meat, none of them contains oils that have a bad effect on the blood. Nuts and seeds can be chopped in a grinder and added to salads, stews, breakfast cereal, or sprinkled over fruit.

For our bodies to function properly we need vitamins and minerals for growth, for repair, to provide energy and strength, to regulate blood sugar and to help our brains to function. To prevent disease and stimulate the production of enzymes we need to take in a whole range of vitamins, which act as catalysts in the body ensuring the production of enzymes that regulate its biochemistry – balancing hormones, producing energy and boosting the immune system. Minerals such as iron, calcium, magnesium, zinc, manganese, chromium, selenium, potassium and phosphorus work, either by themselves or in combination with each other, to ensure healthy cell growth and repair, to control blood sugar levels, to boost the immune system and to provide strength and energy. For example, iron carries the oxygen in the blood, zinc is vital for body repair and renewal and for sexual functioning, selenium and zinc working together help to boost the immune system, and calcium and magnesium working together ensure healthy bones and teeth. Fruit and vegetables, seeds, nuts, lentils, beans and peas can provide all of these essential elements, provided that you make them part of your daily diet.

A word of caution! Consuming handfuls of salted or dry roast peanuts may provide essential minerals and oils but the benefits will be lost because of the salt and other additives, which will rob the nuts of the essential nutrients.

Fats and oils

If you have a diet that is rich in meat, dairy products, cooking oils and fats, your body can easily become saturated with damaging compounds. Animal fats from meat, burgers, dairy products and, nowadays, also from chicken are unhealthy, and these fats can destroy the good fats from plant foods in a way that results in inflammation. The fats contained in animal products are saturated fats. Palm oil and coconut oil also fall into this group of fats. Olive oil, however, is polyunsaturated, which means that it is more likely to have a beneficial effect on the system because it contains omega-3, omega-6 and omega-9 and ensures a healthy balance of fats in the body. This is what the body needs.

None of these oils should be heated to a high level because this alters their structure and they become saturated. Any vegetable oil that is hardened to make margarine also becomes saturated and therefore harmful to the system. Advice on cooking with oil and avoiding the dangers is given in the recipe section (see p. 64).

Water

In reviewing the major elements of diet it is so easy to overlook the importance of water. Our bodies are made up of two-thirds water and we lose 1.5 litres a day through the skin, the lungs and natural elimination via the kidneys. It is recommended that you drink 1–2 litres a day to replace the water lost. A diet rich in vegetables will provide more water than a diet rich in meat, which robs the body of water during the digestive process. The water provided from vegetable intake is easily assimilated by the body and provides a high percentage of vitamins and minerals. If you have up to nine portions of fruit and vegetables a day it is possible to replace half the amount of water needed. This leaves about a litre to be consumed as water, diluted fruit juice, herb teas or fruit teas. Alcohol, tea and coffee cause the body to lose water and as a result deplete the body's minerals.

Essentially, water should be rich in minerals but there is a school of thought that suggests that tap water is depleted in calcium and at the same time carries nitrates, lead and aluminium that limit the nutritional value of our food. Filtering gets rid of the 'baddies' but unfortunately it may also take away some of the essential minerals. The carbon in artificially carbonated bottled water is known to attract the minerals in the body, which are expelled before they can do their work. However, naturally carbonated 'sparkling' water from deep in the earth is rich in minerals and aids your nutrition.

Elimination of water by the kidneys as urine gets rid of toxins from the body. Unfortunately, we can overload our body with toxic material. A diet rich in animal fats and sugars produces too much of a strain on the 'cleansing department' and so toxins are not easily eliminated. Toxins get stored away in the cells in various parts of the body. The situation is made worse when we consume too much refined and processed food that contains nutrient-destroying or useless elements. We also live in a toxic environment, very high in pollutants. All of these things tax the body's ability to cope, and a build-up of toxins is a precursor to the development of allergies and other illnesses.

Adjusting to a new diet

It takes a while to adjust to any new diet, particularly if it means abandoning favourite foods. It took me ages to give up the bacon butty. The smell of frying bacon still drives me mad and produces cravings, but then I think of the way I was and the way I feel now and I do not want to go back to the way I was.

I was recently discussing the problems of a man with multiple sclerosis (MS) who had been advised that a change in diet might help him. He studied the diet sheet he had been given by his therapist and compared it to his usual diet. As he did this he imagined the loss of familiar tastes and textures. The negative thoughts of no longer eating cheese, steak or bacon or of no longer drinking coffee or alcohol were far stronger than the prospect of freedom from pain, freedom of movement and greater enjoyment of life. He could not face the demands being made on him and saw them as a completely radical departure from his habitual comforting range of foods and as too high a price to pay. At this stage there was no way he could even imagine making a start on a new diet. After all, he did not see his illness at this time as being life-threatening, and yet a lifetime of eating the kind of diet he was used to was bound in the end to weaken his system so much that his survival would be threatened. He needed help to take the first step. Fortunately he did and is now making good progress towards remission. In reading this book you may identify closely with him and be equally overwhelmed by the prospect of change. Before you go any further, therefore, just think of one change you could make to your eating habits. I leave the choice to you. I just want you to be as pain-free as possible.

If you have pain then there is even more reason to ensure that you have the most nutritious diet available. The aim of this book is to give you the means of working out for yourself how you can choose a diet to suit you. By that I mean one that does not challenge your immune system and provides maximum nutritional value. The diet must do more than that. It must appeal to you on many levels. It must substantially help to reduce inflammation and pain levels and it must help you to begin the process of healing your digestive system so that you become less sensitive to the food you eat. The recommendations I have made will go a long way towards achieving this goal if you follow them. You may well see results from the change of diet within a week or two and eventually you will come to prefer the new tastes, textures and smells. You will feel so much fitter, have much more energy and less pain, and your general health and appearance will improve beyond measure.

My account of my own development from childhood will give you some idea of the timescale involved in doing the damage. There is no quick fix but the time it takes to bring about improvements is comparatively short when measured against the time it has taken for the problems to build up.

5

Laying the foundations

Parents and children

Reflecting on my own experience as a child has made me realize even more the importance of listening to children and taking note of their likes and dislikes. Children go through stages when they turn up their noses at certain foods but it is important that parents develop the skill of listening to them and observing them closely so that they can distinguish between a child being 'faddy' and one being genuinely repelled by some foods. It was only when I approached the age of 60 that I discovered, from relatives of my mother's generation, that I had not walked until I was three years old. I was a bloated baby and apparently, a few years before the Second World War, I attended hospital, where I was put on a special diet. The details of this diet are lost in the mists of time but I was told that it had something to do with my food being 'too rich'. I know that hospital appointments continued and it was recommended that one of my shoes should be built up. No one could recall which one.

I remember that I suffered joint pains throughout childhood but these were dismissed as 'growing pains'. My teenage career as an athlete was blighted by severe muscle cramps and during these years I experienced the first signs of serious digestive problems. When I first went to school I can remember being violently sick and having severe stomach cramps following birthday parties where things like blancmange and junket were served. (Isn't this common after parties?)

My grandparents, who looked after me for the first 10 years of my life, had a smallholding where they reared hens, geese, ducks and rabbits and grew most of their own vegetables. At that time anyone who reared poultry could exchange their egg ration for animal feed. My mother, who was a widow, was engaged in war service. Twice a day I would go with my grandmother to collect a flagon of full-cream milk from the farm next door. This was made into milky puddings, rice, tapioca and sago and, even though they plainly disagreed with me, I was forced to eat them up as they were 'good for me'! In school I was often sickened by the taste and smell of compulsory school milk, and I can remember feeling heavy and miserable on many occasions after drinking it. Things being 'good for me' was a recurring theme throughout my childhood, and my mother had learned well from my grandmother that same message – 'You must eat it because it is good for you. If you don't you will get ill.' To me this did not make any sense because I knew if I ate it I would feel ill. I am sure I was not alone in this, especially during the war when food was scarce and nothing could be wasted. Children were admonished for not clearing their plates and there were even threats of physical punishment if food was left. We were reminded that 'There is a war on! Think of the starving refugees – and the soldiers in the desert!' We wanted to do our bit – even if it was just to eat up the rice pudding!

These were days of rationing, when children were not asked what they would like to eat. It was an achievement to gather together the ingredients for a meal. There were no supermarkets, only shops selling specific foods so mothers had to queue at the grocer, the greengrocer, the butcher, the dairy, and this could take most of the morning. I can remember helping my grandmother carry heavy shopping bags to our home nearly two miles away. The meal was cooked and everyone was expected to eat and enjoy it. It was a tribute to the love and care that the cook had put into it. It was not just food – it was Mother's food! To leave any on the plate was considered bad manners, an insult to the cook and much worse, a rejection of the parent. Not liking something was no excuse for leaving it. My grandfather frequently reinforced this message and his word could not be questioned. Recognition of food sensitivity was a long way off. It would not have been understood by my grandparents at a point in history when such a diagnosis was unheard of.

There was no point in my complaining that something tasted 'funny', because everyone else at the table had eaten the food and praised it. Wartime government-issue orange juice tasted to me like vinegar and the much-prized chocolate ration had a metallic taste. I could not see how anyone could say they enjoyed it, but I suppose it was much like someone who is colour-blind and naturally assumes that everybody sees the same colours as they do. I was led to believe that when ice-cream was reintroduced after the war, I was in for a major treat and for two or three years looked forward with great anticipation to my first taste but to my horror it tasted more like soap. I had some in the cinema at the Saturday afternoon matinee and my enjoyment of Flash Gordon was completely ruined because I developed a blinding headache. Even though I was unaware that I had a milk allergy, from that day onwards I have never eaten ice-cream in a cinema. With hindsight, my food reactions were probably indicative of a number of food sensitivities, and I would hope that any child growing up now would be observed closely and listened to. In spite of all the signs, the adults would not have accepted for a moment that the food they were lovingly providing for me could possibly harm me in any way.

Skin rashes, lumps, itching, stomach cramps and diarrhoea, recurring joint pains and muscle cramps were not related to food sensitivity; neither were they investigated medically. Stomach ache and vomiting, quite common in young children, were accepted as the result of over-indulgence or eating something that 'disagreed', the remedy for which was Andrews liver salts or milk of magnesia, and aspirin was used liberally as a 'cure-all'. At the age of 18 I experienced my first abdominal bleeding, and it was not until a few years later when I had a further severe bleeding that I was informed I was allergic to aspirin, which had caused ulceration of the stomach – and a milk diet was prescribed!

I use my own case as an example of the importance of listening to children, observing recurrent symptoms and getting the best medical advice.

I make no excuse for introducing an autobiographical chapter at this stage. Part of my quest, which investigated the possibility that food had something to do with my illness, involved a complete examination of my childhood and adolescence. This followed my discovery of the dairy-free cookery book in Canada.

My findings since that time are verified by the work of a number of medical researchers who have investigated this topic. Sensitivity to food from early infancy is the first sign of a disease-making process. If the diet is not corrected at an early stage, then the process towards ill health will continue and a number of chronic symptoms are likely to be triggered throughout life until the person becomes acutely ill. The acute illness phase may only be reached at times of stress or if the lifestyle becomes too hectic or if the person develops an unhealthy eating pattern, perhaps missing meals and making do with a bag of crisps or a burger. I know that my teenage health crisis came when I was studying for A levels and doing a part-time job as a postman during the heaviest snowfall for years. I was skimping on meals because I never had enough time. I was also taking part in cross-country races each weekend in all weathers. I caught flu, took aspirin and within a few days had my first severe haemorrhage. No one was aware that I had a sensitivity to aspirin or that I had had a sensitivity to milk since infancy.

Research has also indicated that a number of inflammatory illnesses have their roots in childhood and can evolve over many years. However, we only seem to take note of acute, major illness and no one seems to link years of suffering many minor chronic symptoms such as sinus problems, muscle aches and pains, headaches, stomach aches, eczema, digestive problems or chronic constipation. A person complaining of these things might be called a hypochondriac. It is these symptoms that ought to be noted as children grow up, otherwise they can build up until life events such as divorce, moving house, an infection, an injury, a drug reaction or childbirth precipitate a major disabling illness. This point is expanded on in Chapter 9, the chapter on stress.

6

Food as an emotional subject rooted in culture and habits

There is a big emotional investment in food, and a child very soon learns that in order to please parents he or she must not only eat what is provided but clear the plate even though the portion size may be out of all proportion to the child's needs. However, the child can also use this complex relationship between food and affection as a weapon against the parent to draw attention. I have seen parents in tears when a child has refused to eat a meal that has taken two hours to prepare. Children can often end up with a very peculiar diet that enables the family to avoid conflict at mealtimes. This makes it very difficult for a parent who has the responsibility for ensuring that the child develops physically and remains healthy and who at the same time must assess what food and how much food will meet the child's needs. Parents also have to cope with cultural pressures, which have a very strong influence on their own habits and their views of what constitutes 'good' food.

In recent years parents have had to incorporate into their children's diets medical opinion about how children should be fed and at the same time make decisions in the light of a welter of advertising. The supermarket shelves are stacked with colourfully packaged foods and only recently has there been an attempt to show the nutritional value of these 'goodies'. The labelling still leaves a lot to be desired, and one needs a degree in nutrition to make sense of it all. Take cows' milk for example. It is not the same product as it was in the past. Milk is now treated to the extent that all the natural healthy bacteria are removed during processing. Cows are fed growth hormones and dosed liberally with antibiotics to counter all the diseases that cattle are heir to, and these hormones and antibiotics are transmitted into the meat and the milk. Knowing this, even if I were not sensitive to dairy produce, I would have excluded milk from choice.

I note from recent government-sponsored reports that allergies and food sensitivities are increasing dramatically throughout the world. This phenomenon is put down to changed 'environmental factors' such as pollutants from diesel fuel, children being brought up in a 'too clean' environment where they are not in contact with germs which play their part in developing the immune system. I think these views need to be challenged. It seems to me too simplistic an answer. Food has changed radically during the last 50 years. Chemicals, preservatives and colorants all play their part in altering food. Even so-called fresh food is being chemically treated. Meat is taken apart in factories and reconstituted in completely different proportions from the original. Then the chemicals are added. This applies to cooked meats and pies as well as re-formed 'joints' of beef, lamb and pork, which are not really joints but simulations made from cheaper cuts of meat.

It has only recently been officially accepted that cocktails of additives, particularly colorants, can adversely affect the behaviour of children, even though attention was drawn to this problem some years ago, and concern has been expressed that additives, approved only because they are not 'poisonous', contribute to the depletion of nutrients in the body. I await the results of further research on the effects of other food additives on the growing number of allergies and food sensitivities that are being experienced by the population.

Although the British have embraced the cuisines of Italy, China, Thailand and India, and relish the high-fat fast foods, potato crisps and sugary drinks of the USA, they still hold on to old habits and to the sort of food that their grandparents might have eaten while they were working in the fields or factories. They find it difficult to contemplate giving up tea, coffee, bread, pies, pasties, joints of meat, sausages, bacon, and fish and chips. With increased affluence and cheaper foods, people can afford to indulge themselves much more than our grandparents could, without doing the same amount of physical work or walking the same distances. I was recently in the company of someone who claimed that for almost every Saturday of his 60 years of marriage he and his wife had enjoyed meat pies from the same shop. It was a ritual that he would never consider giving up. Even although he and his wife have reached a ripe old age, they stumble from one hospital appointment to another with a whole range of chronic illness. I would not say the pies had added anything to their enjoyment of old age.

Some people manage to avoid fruit and vegetables altogether and anyone who departs from the cultural norms is considered to be faddy or half-starved or to have no appreciation of 'good food'.

The UK shares a wider northern European culture where there is an emphasis on maintaining a thriving dairy industry. There is always a plentiful supply of milk, cheese, butter and meat. Individual governments and the European Union have devoted a large amount of taxpayers' money in subsidies to maintain this industry.

In the second half of the twentieth century the British government and health professionals extolled the virtues of cows' milk as essential for healthy growth and development. I can remember when I was nine years old being addressed at school by a visitor from some government organization exhorting the children to drink milk. She displayed many pictures and charts showing the difference between children who did not drink milk and those who did. Needless to say, the ones who drank milk had rosy complexions and were seen enjoying many physical activities. The non-milk drinkers were shown as puny and lethargic. This was justified at the time because of the history of malnutrition and its attendant illnesses, such as rickets and tuberculosis, among the poor. Milk was seen as the prime source of protein and calcium.

Nowadays this blind allegiance to dairy produce is inappropriate. There is a view that cows' milk should not be fed to any species other than cattle, including humans – on the grounds that human digestion cannot cope with it. It is thought that cows' milk might be playing a part in contributing to the high incidence of obesity, heart disease, diabetes and other illnesses. We have had no recent official pronouncements on the value of dairy products in the diet but it is noticeable that skimmed and semi-skimmed milk are promoted commercially, and there are warnings about a high intake of animal fats. There is now not so much emphasis on the importance of drinking milk, but it is difficult to avoid feeding children with over-abundant levels of sugar-loaded yoghurts and milky desserts, ice-cream, fruity milk-based drinks and many products bulked out with milk protein, milk powder, whey, caseinates and lactose. It is now impossible to measure how much milk and dairy fat a child is consuming.

All of these products are backed up by expensive television advertising that encourages children to pester their parents into buying the latest desserts or drinks. Because parents have been encouraged over the years to be anxious about the development of their children, they are easily persuaded that giving in is a good thing for the health of their children, and at the same time a way of keeping them quiet.

It is quite surprising to go to southern Europe and find that people live and eat quite differently, consuming a wide variety of fish, olive oil, fruit and vegetables, and salads. No doubt in these countries the cultural reinforcements for this diet are just as strong as they are in the UK. Wherever you are in the world food has an emotional and social importance over and above its nutritional value.

For example, at Christmas the celebrations involve eating specific foods in the company of members of the family. People will go to great inconvenience and expense to be 'home' in time for Christmas dinner. I am prompted to think that the whole period should perhaps be renamed 'Kill a Granny Week'. Either granny stays at home and cooks for a dozen or more even though she may not be physically up to it, or she is expected to accept an invitation from some of the family to travel many miles in the middle of winter, just so that she will not have her Christmas dinner alone. One Christmas while waiting for friends at a crowded Waverley Station in Edinburgh, we witnessed a number of agitated elderly women struggling alone through the milling crowds with large suitcases, no doubt full of presents, to find their carriage and then their reserved seat on a train to London, only to find that because of service problems none of the seats bore the correct reservation tickets. They might just as well have been asked to take part in a rugby match! This is an example of the emotional investment that families put on that particular meal. I have no doubt that the Americans have a similar investment in Thanksgiving and that the Spanish, French or Italians place similar importance in being home for their numerous religious festivals, when families and their communities come together to enjoy a feast.

My story has illustrated how difficult it is to step outside the cultural or family values so far as food is concerned. There are many pressures on people to conform – from parents, friends, family, workmates and the culture in general. It is very difficult in the UK to avoid 'chips with everything' when eating out and, if you do, you do so at a price.

I was talking to a German friend recently about food and food sensitivities and he claimed he would be ill if he did not eat meat every day. He could not imagine a life without meat. The meat he was talking about was what I call strong meat: beefsteak, lamb or pork. To him vegetables were just a garnish and not really valued for themselves. He reckoned his diet did him no harm whatsoever, yet he had a heart problem and high blood pressure.

Your body, your food, your health . . .

Unfortunately, we are eating more food than ever before. Portions are so much larger, and whole evenings can be spent in front of the TV snacking and drinking. As a result we are consuming more saturated fat and sugar in our diet. However, when people try to exercise individual choice in their diet, as do vegetarians or vegans or people with food sensitivities, they are often treated as being odd or 'faddy'. Twenty years ago I remember being concerned when my two sons, who by then were living away from home, embraced the vegetarian message. I felt strongly that without meat or fish they would not get the best nutritional value from their food, but I was wrong. Even now it is difficult to find a restaurant that caters particularly for vegetarians or vegans, and in most restaurants where concessions are made there is very little real choice.

The attitude to food intolerance seems ambivalent. Newspapers may carry articles highlighting the increase in food allergy and food intolerance, and the same newspapers may also have scathing articles about the 'imagined' allergies that people claim to have and to relate these to the various food fads that allegedly originate in California. Do not be put off by those who scorn the idea of a 'choosy' diet, saying it is just a fad. People might say, 'I can eat anything. It has never done me any harm.' Just pause a little and consider, are these people on tablets for blood pressure or diabetes or are they overweight or even obese?

You do not have to tell anyone about your food preference unless they are actually preparing a meal for you. It is a matter for your personal concern. However, many people with food sensitivities will continue to eat what is placed before them in the family or when visiting a friend lest they offend, and they may be prepared to suffer extremely uncomfortable consequences. I interviewed a woman recently about the problems she experienced as someone who has been diagnosed with coeliac disease. This disorder arises from an inability of the body to digest gluten, an ingredient that is found particularly in wheat and that makes wheat suitable for making bread and cakes because of its 'sticky' quality. People with coeliac disease will suffer very severe symptoms – mainly loss of weight, bloating, stomach and bowel pains, depression and mood swings – and will generally suffer the consequences of being unable to assimilate nutrients from their diet. The only remedy for this problem is to avoid all products that may contain wheat and gluten. I was concerned to find out how she managed when eating out, visiting friends or going on holiday. It was interesting that this middle-aged person, having been aware of the problem since her teenage years, said that she very rarely ate out and would not go on holiday unless it was self-catering. When visiting friends, they did not always provide the right meals for her but, rather than offend them, she ate what was on offer. Similarly, if she had to eat at a restaurant and there was nothing suitable on the menu she generally accepted what she thought would do the least harm and was then prepared to suffer the consequences for the next week or two. Unfortunately, people with coeliac problems can, if the diet is neglected, develop arthritis – an additional burden to cope with.

In spite of all the pressures that people experience over the question of food, they still make their own choices about what they feel is good for them. These choices are based not so much on nutritional value but on the senses – sight, taste and smell – so some people might choose not to eat vegetables at all and have a diet based on high-fat foods and fizzy drinks. Others may choose not to take cheese or milk because they do not like the smell or because it makes them feel queasy, causes catarrh or gives them bad dreams. They would not accept that they have a food intolerance. They may blame the discomfort on other factors or resort to indigestion tablets and nasal inhalers. Some choose not to eat strawberries because they get a rash or their digestive system becomes sore. You may be one of the many who do not drink tea because the tannins and acidity give you indigestion. Or again, you may drink it and pop in an antacid tablet. There are many who do not eat fried food or pastry because it is hard to digest. When I was a child I was amazed when I visited the home of a distant relative whose son, on his return home from work, sat down to an enormous plate of potatoes and nothing else. Some people will never eat fish unless it is hidden in batter and covered in chips. Many will refuse all seafood because they cannot bear the thought of eating it. I can remember my grandparents giving me tripe to eat. I had never eaten it before and had no preconceived ideas about it but at the first mouthful I was sick. Look around your family and think about the likes and dislikes of each member. As you will see, there is no 'one size fits all' diet. We make choices about the things we eat for many reasons, and not all of our choices bring nutritional benefits.

Comfort eating plays a major part in our choice of food at times of stress, when there are relationship problems and when we are bored or generally feeling unloved or undervalued. Like others with chronic pain, I have sought comfort in food and as a result have put on weight, which added to my problems. In a later chapter I shall explore this point in greater depth when I consider the concepts of stress, chronic pain, diet and food sensitivity (see Chapters 7, 8 and 9).

We need to be much more rational in our choices of food, basing our choice on its nutritional and healing value. It is my aim in the next few chapters to show how this can be done in order to limit your pain and heal your body.

In the past, the ingredients of a meal in any culture were determined by what was available locally. It is only in recent years that a global cuisine has developed where food is available from all over the world at almost any time of year.

Following that chance reading of the cookery book in the Toronto bookshop, I cut out cows' milk and went over to soya and rice milks. Almost at once I experienced relief from the asthma attacks, the tingling of the lips, the wheezing, the soreness of the throat and the feeling that my digestive tract had been stripped of its lining.

If you are new to the whole question of how food affects the body, it is easy to get confused by some of the terms that are used by journalists, the medical profession, nutritionists and other people who profess to have some knowledge of the subject. Even professionals seem to get technical terms muddled and in the same article: having gone to great lengths to identify the difference between a food allergy and food intolerance, they will go on to talk of allergies as embracing all types of reaction to food.

7

What does it mean to be allergic, intolerant or sensitive to food?

All three reactions to food – allergy, intolerance and sensitivity – can be equally distressing to the sufferer, but there are differences that need to be understood, especially as further on in this chapter I talk about foods that can be triggers for your pain.

Food sensitivity

Food sensitivity is a term that covers any adverse reaction to a food or a chemical, which may occur naturally in a food or which may be added to a food as a preservative, a colouring, an emulsifier, a thickener or a bulking agent. Under the umbrella of 'food sensitivity' are included the terms 'food allergy' and 'food intolerance'. Pain may be triggered by any food sensitivity, whether it is defined as an allergy or an intolerance.

Food allergy

A food allergy is a reaction to certain foods, producing symptoms that can occur within minutes of eating the food or, in extreme cases, after touching or even smelling it. The symptoms can be severe and commonly include asthma attacks, nausea and vomiting, swelling and skin rashes, runny eyes and nose, eczema, severe headaches, urticaria (hives) and, in the most extreme cases, anaphylactic shock (causing a total collapse and, in rare instances, death). It seems in the case of allergies, the body is unable to digest the protein that causes the problem and the protein is allowed to pass directly into the bloodstream. The body recognizes this protein as an intruder or antigen and produces antibodies, usually referred to as immunoglobin E. As this travels round the body cells called mast cells open to release histamines into the bloodstream, and these histamines produce the allergic reaction and cause an inflammatory response. This inflammatory response is what causes the symptoms. The most common culprits associated with food allergy include:

- cows' milk and anything made from it;
- eggs;
- nuts;
- fish and seafood;
- wheat and gluten (a person can be sensitive to wheat but not to gluten – if you are sensitive to wheat only then you can eat oats, barley and rye);
- chocolate.

There are other food items to which people are allergic, including:

- corn;
- alcohol;
- strawberries;
- chemicals that may be used in processed foods and also in medicines.

It is usually recommended that anyone with a food allergy should take steps to avoid eating the offending food.

Food intolerance

Food intolerances are more common than food allergies. Although they are abnormal reactions to food, or chemicals within the food, they do not involve the immune system – unlike allergies. Whatever the definition and whether your immune system is involved or not, the symptoms of both can be extremely unpleasant and have the potential to limit severely your quality of life.

Recognizing food sensitivities

Food allergy can usually be diagnosed by means of a case history and skin and blood tests. There will probably be evidence of the antigens and their antibodies in the samples, but the tests are not always reliable and can produce a false-negative result.

Tests for food intolerance are much more problematic, and they can be inconvenient and distressing, involving a lengthy investigation. To achieve an effective diagnosis it is necessary to remove potential suspect foods from the diet for a few weeks at a time. If there is an absence of symptoms during the elimination period then the diagnosis of food intolerance can be confirmed. However, the symptoms may not disappear and other foods might have to be eliminated in turn until the culprit is found. To confirm the diagnosis, the food is then reintroduced gradually in order to see if the symptoms recur. It is recommended that such an elimination diet should only be attempted with appropriate medical supervision. There is concern that imposing any restriction on the diet may severely compromise its nutritional value, and the process may take several weeks for all the suspect foods to be tested. I have some reservations about the logic of this. If you have a food intolerance and experience all the accompanying discomfort and upset in your body then it is likely that your nutrition is already compromised. Whenever I have sought medical advice on the subject of food intolerance, the response has been either to accept my word that a particular food is causing me a problem – and I have been advised to eliminate it from my diet – or there has been a suggestion that if I know what is bothering me it is hardly worth going to the trouble of having a test! As there are only a handful of centres specializing in the subject, this suggestion has presumably been made because of the lack of facilities.

Over the years I have learned to 'listen' to my body. I have a good inner sense of what makes me feel good and of those things that have the opposite effect. One advantage of having a chronic pain problem is that the pain itself has become a barometer for indicating the 'goodies' and 'baddies' in my diet. If I have taken in something to which I am sensitive, for instance animal fat, within a very short time I get a strong pain in the middle of my back (always in the same place). If I take in wheat or gluten I experience muscle weakness within minutes. My walking is affected and my overall pain level increases. Over the next few days I then feel intense depression and experience bloating and severe constipation. It takes at least a week for the symptoms to ease. Milk is easily recognized. Initially my lips start to tingle, my mouth becomes swollen and my airways also swell so that I have difficulty breathing and also find myself choking. Eventually, I get a sore throat and it feels as though the lining has been stripped from my digestive tract. Again, it can take several days for these symptoms to move unless of course I take emergency action, which fortunately helps to shorten the reaction time.

It may be that people with chronic pain have never related their pain level to food that they have ingested but put it down to other factors – the weather, standing too long, sitting too long, not sleeping well; the list is endless.

If I suspect that a particular food is causing me problems, I cut it out for 10 days before trying it again, and if I then experience the same symptoms I eliminate the food again, for good this time – unless of course I accidentally consume the offending food; then the uncomfortable symptoms recur. The situation is further complicated by the fact that a particular food may not always produce a bad reaction and the reaction may depend on the frequency or amount of that food that you eat. The response may depend on other factors such as tiredness or stress, so that symptoms may occur some times and not others. This adds to the difficulty of diagnosis.

Eliminating foods without eliminating nutrients

Having gone through this process several times I was concerned that I may not be getting sufficient nourishment from my food. As a result of eliminating foods that were causing me problems (pain, bowel problems, muscle weakness, fatigue and sleeplessness), I concluded that whatever I was now eating was making me feel much better because most of my problems had cleared up, including the frequency and intensity of pain. However, I did seek the advice of a nutritionist and underwent a number of tests that have been clinically tested and approved in the USA. It was most helpful to me in making my own decisions in working out a diet that was nourishing and trouble-free.

Put simply, the tests that I was given are based on the theory that every food and chemical has an electrical signature to which the body reacts either positively or negatively. They involved being linked by an electrode to a computer. The body's reaction to an electrical impulse too small to cause any discomfort is measured, and the strength of the reaction indicates the degree of sensitivity a person has to a particular food or chemical. I have no wish to enter into the debate on the reliability of these tests but Eve and I have both undertaken the test, which is known as electrodermal screening. It is non-invasive and provides information designed to give a clearer understanding of a person's health. I undertook the test knowing that I had a number of food sensitivities, and my main concern was to find out which foods were the most appropriate for me to eat. As I was rather sceptical about non-NHS approved tests, Eve also undertook the test as a control because, to her knowledge, there were no foods to which she was sensitive. In my case the test confirmed my sensitivity to those foods I knew affected me but the results indicated there were other foods

I should eat with caution. The nutritionist was able to advise which foods should be avoided altogether and those that should be eaten infrequently and in small amounts.

Over a period of time, as the body adjusted to being without the offending foods, further testing by the same method showed that foods that had previously figured as suspect in the original test had become more acceptable to my body. Consequently I was able to increase the range of foods available to me. As an example, potatoes were placed on a list of foods to be eaten with caution, no more than once a month or so. My experience tallies with the accepted idea that the severity of symptoms in some cases of food intolerance is dependent on the quantity you eat and how often you have it. I find that if I eat potatoes too often, and in quantity, then I experience digestive problems and my pain problem increases over a period of a few days.

Eve's test confirmed that she had little to worry about as far as her food intake was concerned but the nutritionist was able to make suggestions relating to some of her favourite foods, over-consumption of which might eventually lead to food sensitivities. Such sensitivities may be said to be 'dormant' at the moment but continued overuse, combined with a period of stress, might bring the sensitivities to the fore. These dormant sensitivities mainly involved foods that she was particularly fond of – oranges, tomatoes and wholemeal bread, which she had eaten all her life, on a daily basis. It is not necessarily new foods that trigger sensitivities. Sometimes the body will reject a food that you have eaten all your life, for no apparent reason.

Anyone at any age can develop bad reactions to foods or to chemicals that are added to food. For example, older people often develop an intolerance of milk and milk products, having consumed them throughout their lives. People who have eaten a food for so long are often very resistant to the idea that it is causing them any harm. In my experience, just as tastes change over the years, so our body's reactions also change. It may be that, with age, our ability to absorb certain foods diminishes and that enzymes responsible for the digestion of fats or carbohydrates are either absent or weakened. In the case of dairy produce it is suggested that the absence of an enzyme called lactase makes it impossible for the body to assimilate lactose, which is present in cows' milk.

The symptoms of food intolerance may not occur immediately after the offending food has been consumed. This is in contrast to food allergy, where there is usually an immediate reaction. It may take anything up to four or five days for symptoms to appear and this makes it difficult to pin down the culprit. Although we can be intolerant of virtually anything in our diet, it is generally accepted that the main foods which cause reactions are wheat, corn, dairy produce, tomatoes, potatoes, eggs, nuts, sulphites and nitrites (which are often added to food as a preservative and are found in wine, cooked meats, bacon and sausages).

A word of caution! Many of the symptoms of food allergy and food intolerance may be caused by other problems, so do not always assume that your symptoms result from food sensitivity. If your symptoms are of recent onset then it is important that you seek medical advice and have a thorough check-up. It is important that any suspicions of food sensitivity are followed up. If you continue to consume food that produces bad reactions, you not only have to cope with recurring discomfort but you will not be getting nutritional benefits and you may even be suffering from cumulative digestive and intestinal damage, which will add to the stress you are already suffering as a result of your pain. In Chapter 9 I look in much more detail at the whole question of stress and its relationship to food sensitivity and pain.

Although clearly it is sensible to exclude any foods to which you are allergic or sensitive, you should also take steps to see whether the problem of food sensitivity can be tackled at its source. If your body is recognizing certain foods as 'enemy invaders' then there is obviously something wrong in your digestive system that needs to be fixed. The purpose of the digestive system is to digest food in such a way that the nutrients can be distributed around your body to nourish the cells. Improperly absorbed food will lead to many other problems, and the likelihood is that the sensitivities and the accompanying symptoms will increase. When a food, such as wheat, irritates your system and is not fully absorbed, your immune system is challenged constantly if you continue to eat that food. Your digestive system is left with the problem of dealing with the undigested or partially digested food. Continued intake of the offending food may eventually weaken the immune system and possibly lead to even more serious problems. When eating an offending food for the first time you may just experience mild discomforts such as catarrh or bloating, but if the problem is not identified early you may experience allergic reactions, for example to gluten, which may mean avoiding this substance for the rest of your life.

8

Foods that can spell danger!

Do any of these foods trigger your pain?

Since the beginning of the 1980s, research has focused on specific trigger foods. These foods are harmless to most people but a minority of people may be particularly sensitive to one or more of them. Although problem foods vary from person to person, it is now known that specific foods are associated with painful conditions and inflammation. These are known as trigger foods.

The major trigger foods are:

- dairy products, including milk, cream, ice-cream, yoghurt, whey, butter and cheese;
- corn;
- all meats;
- fish;
- wheat, oats and rye;
- eggs;
- citrus fruits;
- potatoes, tomatoes, capsicums (sweet peppers) – all members of the deadly nightshade family;
- nuts;
- coffee;
- alcohol;
- chocolate.

For some reason the researchers have not included tea in their list of trigger foods, but I think it is important to highlight some of the issues surrounding tea in relation to its role in exacerbating pain conditions. Anyone with pain should be aware that tea (and by this I mean black tea, which is the most popular variety drunk in the UK) is fermented after it has been picked and before it is dried. As a result of this treatment, the tea is high in tannic acid, which can irritate the lining of the stomach and cause inflammation. Anything that increases inflammation in the body should be avoided by people with an inflammatory illness. A distinction needs to be made between black, fermented tea and green and other teas that do not undergo fermentation and, as a result, are not high in tannins; neither do such teas contain caffeine.

Coffee is also high in acidity and can bring about stomach irritation and inflammation, particularly when numerous cups are drunk each day. Many people seek safety in drinking decaffeinated coffee but the decaffeination process does nothing to reduce the acidity, and the chemicals used in the process can also cause problems for people with pain.

Caffeine, found in tea, coffee and other drinks such as colas, and in some medicines, heightens sensitivity, and no one with pain needs this.

Food additives

Food additives contain elements that contribute to hormone imbalances that may be responsible for joint pain and other health problems. The problem is for each individual to explore which of these foods are triggers. Fortunately, we do not have to start from scratch in our attempts to find out what these are, since they are well documented: research shows that pain, discomfort and deterioration in function in a number of conditions are triggered by the same group of foods. These conditions are osteoarthritis, rheumatoid arthritis, multiple sclerosis, fibromyalgia, and migraine and other recurring headaches. Below are given some examples of the effects of food on these illnesses.

Arthritis

Many people who have rheumatoid arthritis or osteoarthritis are known to be sensitive to wheat and dairy produce. In fact most chronic pain problems are aggravated by too much refined sugar, by stimulants, by animal fats and by too much protein. It is worthwhile for anyone with pain to get used to a diet that excludes red meat, all dairy produce, alcohol, tea and coffee. Citrus fruits, which are also on the list of trigger foods, should be avoided.

Fibromyalgia

This debilitating condition is very difficult to diagnose. Its symptoms are very similar to myalgic encephalopathy (ME) or chronic fatigue syndrome. However, anyone who has fibromyalgia is clearly suffering from chronic pain. The illness is not clearly understood, and people with fibromyalgia may feel they are being dismissed by the medical profession on the grounds that the problems are imagined. The result is that sufferers are often treated inappropriately with antidepressants or tranquillizers.

Signs and symptoms of the illness can change from one day to the next. Pain can move from one limb to another and from one side of the body to the other. Pain can be at many sites of the body but it is accepted that people with fibromyalgia have chronic muscular, joint and tendon pain along with extreme fatigue. Unlike arthritic problems, it is not usual for there to be signs of inflammation, redness, heat or deformity. It is thought that the illness usually follows the stress of physical or psychological trauma, surgery or infection.

It is known that people with fibromyalgia respond mostly to progressive physical exercise, relaxation and a good diet. The dietary aspect is discussed below (see p. 43), but it is known that things to be avoided are alcohol, tea, coffee, fizzy drinks, refined sugar and even fish. Research has indicated that sulphites used as preservatives and added to red wines, cooked meats and many other foods can act as triggers, along with dairy products, corn and some fruits. Avoiding these foods can bring about significant improvements in the pain of fibromyalgia.

It is suggested, as a result of clinical studies, that regular exercise is extremely important in reducing pain, sensitivity to touch, and fatigue. It also helps to alleviate depression and to improve bowel symptoms. This is true for most chronic pain conditions, and it is worth repeating it here. In addition to the food sensitivities mentioned, people with fibromyalgia have been found to have significantly low levels of magnesium in their system, and boosting this mineral, along with calcium, can also bring about improvement.

Migraine

It is now commonly accepted that up to 50 per cent of people who regularly suffer from migraine improve when trigger foods are removed from their diet. A person may respond badly to a single food, but migraine can often be triggered by a number of foods. These can be foods that a person likes best. In my experience people never seem to accept that a food that they like a lot can possibly do them any harm – but the reverse is often true. Any of the foods on the trigger list at the beginning of this chapter can set off an episode but there are others such as onions and bananas that are known also to trigger migraines.

Foods that are considered safe

However, foods can also work towards restoring the hormone balance and therefore controlling the inflammatory response. Foods that are considered safe, producing few, if any, problems and working towards restoring the balance are:

- brown rice;
- cooked or dried fruits (but beware of additives such as sulphur dioxide), though not citrus fruit, kiwi fruit, bananas, peaches or tomatoes;
- all vegetables, but go easy on potatoes; focus mainly on green leafy vegetables, cabbage, spring greens, spinach, broccoli, artichokes, asparagus, carrots, parsnips.

Food additives and your pain

In the past 50 years, many more additives, derived from natural or chemical sources, have been introduced to food. Throughout the world these additives are assigned numbers, and in Europe each of the numbers is prefixed by 'E' to signify that they are approved for use within Europe. They are used as preservatives, bulking agents, food colourings, colour retention agents and emulsifiers (which enable oils and water to mix, as in mayonnaise). Many food manufacturers use flavour enhancers or flour treatment agents to improve the colour of the flour or its performance in baking. Thickeners are added to liquids; anti-caking agents stop powders clogging and make them flow more easily; preservatives inhibit moulds and contamination by bacteria. Not all of these additives are bad, and they have extended the range of foods available to us throughout the whole year instead of just a short season.

Most food additives are considered to be safe – that is, not poisonous to humans when small quantities are added to food. There are worries, however, that because they are used in so many foods they could build up to toxic levels in the body, especially because some of them used in quantity are known to be carcinogenic. Many people find that they are triggers for allergies, asthma and migraine and that they aggravate chronic pain. It is for this reason that I do not recommend a diet based mainly on processed food – that is, food that has undergone some sort of modification or processing. As you read on you will see that many of the chemicals referred to are likely to cause irritation to the gut or to produce feelings of unease throughout the system. This is particularly important for people who may be on anti-inflammatory drugs, whether prescribed or over-the-counter such as aspirin or ibuprofen, since these drugs are also stomach irritants. It seems silly to exacerbate the problem further by taking in foods that are also irritants. People with pain have enough to cope with without increasing their stress and the likelihood of creating more serious problems.

I know that I respond badly to sulphur dioxide, monosodium glutamate (MSG), sodium metabisulphite, nitrites and sulphites in general. Sulphur dioxide is commonly used to preserve colour in pre-packed meat products and in dried fruit (it is what makes dried apricots orange!). Sulphur dioxide is also added to wine along with sodium metabisulphite as a mould inhibitor. You may be fond of a glass of wine but wine is known to be a trigger for a number of chronic pain conditions and is better avoided if you suspect it is causing you problems. I have found that alcohol in general does not agree with me but in certain situations I can drink red wine without any problem so long as I do not over-indulge. I have very little trouble in France when drinking local young wines but invariably have trouble when I drink wine that has been imported into the UK. For the past couple of years wine bottle labels have carried the words 'contains sulphites', but there is no indication how much. It is inevitable that all wines made from grapes contain a certain level of naturally produced sulphites, which are produced during fermentation. Most countries, including members of the European Union, have agreed that a certain level of sulphites can be added to wine. Sulphites, acting as a mould inhibitor, prevent further fermentation and preserve the wine for much longer periods – very convenient for wine merchants and supermarkets, who want a longer shelf life! However, people like myself suffer the consequences. Sulphites can produce headaches and trigger migraines and can cause itching and skin rashes, and, of course, they are stomach irritants.

In February 2007 the *Seattle Times* reported that consumer groups were lobbying the US Congress about the levels of chemicals being added to wine, citing as an example not only sulphites but colorants especially manufactured for the sole purpose of imparting a deeper red colour so that lesser-quality wines from the final pressings would look more attractive and perhaps seem to be of better quality. The newspaper also reported that a paste made from wheat was being used to fill in the cracks between the planks of the oak barrels to prevent leakage – not good news for people with gluten and wheat allergies. The paper reported that demands were being made for wine to be brought into line with other foodstuffs and that full labelling of all ingredients should be included on bottles. For some reason the trade organizations are not happy about this! The following quotation from the *Seattle Times* from an article by Corrie Brown of the *Los Angeles Times* epitomizes views of many in the wine industry on the subject of honest labelling:

'Why freak out the ignorant when we are adjusting something that is already there in the wine?' says Clark Smith, Chairman of Vinovation, a wine industry 'fix it' shop based in Sebastopol, California. Smith uses additives of all kinds to enhance color and flavour to turn unsuccessful batches of wine from his 1200 winery clients into saleable products. Smith says most of his clients don't share his attitude of openness and he sees no harm in keeping customers in the dark.

Sulphites are used extensively to sterilize equipment in food factories and bottling plants and to prevent apples and potatoes from going brown. Sulphur dioxide E220, when used to bleach flour, destroys most of the vitamin E content. It has a positive function in stabilizing Vitamin C in food but destroys vitamin B1. It can cause gastric irritation and problems for asthma sufferers.

I list below some of the chemicals that are added in order to colour food such as jams, jellies, ice-cream, sauces, cakes, cake mixes, coffee whiteners, yoghurt, fizzy drinks, squashes, marzipan, smoked haddock and kippers.

- E102 tartrazine
- E104 quinoline yellow
- E110 sunshine yellow
- E122 carmoisine
- E124 ponceau 4R
- E127 erithosine
- E128 red 2G
- E131 patent blue V
- E132 indigo carmine
- E133 brilliant blue FCF
- E151 black PN
- E154 brown FK

All these colorants can pose problems for people with food sensitivities and pain. For example, quinoline, which gives a lovely golden colour to smoked haddock, can trigger an inflammatory response, and brown FK, the agent used to make kippers brown, causes a most unpleasant reaction to anyone who is sensitive to aspirin or who has digestive problems or an inflammatory illness – it produces inflammation and water retention and swelling, putting additional stress on the body. As a result it can increase the level of tension and pain. Whenever I have taken brown FK accidentally it has caused acute discomfort for more than a week and I have had to give up normal activity until it has cleared from my system. (Note that naturally smoked products do not contain brown FK.)

All of the colourings mentioned above are used singly or in combination in jams, tinned peas, biscuits, scotch eggs, ice-cream, sausages and garlic sausage, milk shakes, and glacé and cocktail cherries. They can in addition produce adverse reactions such as enlargement of the thyroid gland, sensitivity to light, nausea, low blood pressure, skin sensitivity and itching.

There is a group of additives numbered from E211 to E219. This is the benzoate group of preservatives, which inhibit the growth of yeasts and moulds. Benzoates are used in pie fillings, jams, salad cream, soft drinks, pickles and beer. They can produce unpleasant skin reactions, cause gut irritation and be harmful to people who are sensitive to aspirin. They have also been known to trigger asthma and eczema.

If you have a pain problem you need to beware of E621 – monosodium glutamate – a wheat derivative favoured by Chinese restaurants, take-away food shops and manufacturers of processed food as an additive to enhance the flavour of the food. It appears to stimulate nerve endings and has been responsible for a number of symptoms: hot flushes, headaches, nausea, dizziness and chest pain. It is a well-known migraine trigger and it is not good for people with a wheat or gluten problem.

This is only a brief survey of the whole subject of food additives. Use it as a guide when shopping. It is useful to carry an E numbers pocketbook when you go shopping, since this will give much more information to help you to avoid accidentally buying foods with suspect ingredients. It is normal to print just the E number on labels, and this is where your book will help. It is possible to find processed foods that are safe and contain no suspect additives but you will have to read the labels.

9

Stress

The key to our understanding of the relationship between food sensitivities and chronic pain

Somehow, stress seems to be blamed for anything that goes wrong – for marriage problems, for inability to control children, for lateness at work, for problems with meeting deadlines, for bad manners and for many kinds of unacceptable behaviour. It is used so much and by so many people that its real meaning has become obscured. Just the other day while visiting the Lake District, we walked behind a family on the way back from Windermere to the car park. One of the children, aged about six, had fallen in the water and soaked his trousers. His mother had removed them and he was walking along pulling down his T-shirt to cover his embarrassment. The group met up with some friends and the adults turned all their attention to the newcomers. Suddenly the six-year-old wailed, 'I am having a crisis here. Is no one interested? I am really stressed out!'

Stress is an important medical and psychological term that is crucial in providing a means of understanding the link between illness, chronic pain and diet. Let me explain.

It is generally accepted that the mind and emotions influence the body and physical health. However, not so long ago the Western belief system supported by philosophers and scientists postulated that the mind and the body live in separate compartments and that a person is made up only of physical and chemical reactions, all of which can be measured and manipulated scientifically. For about 200 years the study of the mind and emotions, and their effects on the body, was neglected. However, at the beginning of the last century, Walter Cannon, a physiologist, coined the term 'fight or flight' response for the body's reaction to threats – a quickening of the heart rate, raised blood pressure, change in blood sugar levels, increased muscle tension and faster and more shallow breathing. (This is a very primitive response. I remember the feelings well, occurring at the moment of stepping on to an empty stage to appear in front of a large audience.) At this point our bodies release adrenaline and other chemicals to make us more alert, to raise the blood pressure and to increase strength, speed and reaction time. This response is often the mechanism that comes into play when you hear of acts of bravery. It is very positive, and stress is being used very effectively to achieve some short-term goal. However, problems arise when the stressing event continues for a long period of time. It is difficult for the body to continue working under stress and to continue producing adrenaline without showing signs of protest.

During the 1950s Hans Seyle, researching what he called 'stress', argued that the 'fight or flight' response could be triggered by physiological and psychological factors as well as by physical threats. Within his definition of stress, he maintained that 'fight or flight' reactions can occur where there is no immediate threat except that imagined by a person or stimulated by worry. His work laid the foundation for others to research the relationship between stress and the reactions to it, and the role that these reactions play as causative factors in disease and health and well-being. Whatever the cause of stress – and this can include the experience of long-term illness or pain – the brain reacts by initiating many hundreds of different responses, including the release of a 'cocktail' of chemicals into the bloodstream. Temporarily, these help the person to do what is needed in order to survive. In extreme circumstances, if these chemicals continue to be released the person can experience many adverse changes to behaviour and health. The person might get depressed, find it difficult to sleep, misuse alcohol, experience chest pains and lose immunity to fight disease. Ultimately, the person might succumb to a heart attack or stroke or even die of diseases such as cancer. Seyle, in researching the complex ways in which the mind and body interact, showed how the nervous system works closely with the immune system.

Studies have also shown that thought and emotions can influence the activity of the immune system. When I was a student over 50 years ago, I learned about the general adaptation syndrome (GAS), which is a very useful concept in helping to understand the interaction between stress and the body's reaction to it. At that time I was more interested in the psychological aspects of stress and was given to understand that it was possible for a person to experience a certain level of stress for a considerable time as long as other aspects of life were proceeding well, and that the danger from stress really occurred if the person had to face an additional stress, such as that caused by a sudden bereavement or having to cope with serious illness in the family. I want to go a little bit further in discussing the GAS because I think it is important to understand it fully.

The first stage of the GAS is the alarm reaction – in other words, the previously mentioned 'fight or flight' response, nature's way of protection if something terrible seems to be about to happen. If the cause of stress is removed, the body returns to normal, the heart rate slows down, the breathing rate slows down and the clenched stomach muscles can ease off. If the stress continues, the adaptive process (GAS) goes to the next stage – resistance or adaptation. This is the body's attempt to provide protection over a longer term. More hormones are released, increasing blood sugar levels in order to maintain energy while the person deals with the problem. If this phase continues for a long time and there are no periods of relaxation and rest, the person becomes fatigued. In the effort to sustain high energy levels, coping mechanisms are overtaxed and the person suffers lapses of concentration and may become irritable and lethargic. There is a likelihood at this stage that blood pressure is raised, and eventually a disease process may be initiated when the third stage of the GAS – exhaustion – is reached. At this point the body has run out of reserves, mental, physical and emotional. The body experiences adrenal exhaustion. Blood sugar levels decrease as adrenaline is depleted, leading to decreased stress tolerance and progressive mental and physical exhaustion, and culminating in illness and collapse.

Stress and illness

Virtually any system of the body can exhibit illness as a result of stress. It would be inappropriate to discuss every illness involved, but I should like to focus on those likely to result in chronic pain. The central nervous system may respond to stress by producing anxiety, depression and fatigue. The musculoskeletal system may respond to stress by producing tension in muscles and joints, leading to back problems and muscular aches and pains. Stress, it is suggested, can provoke various degenerative illnesses such as rheumatoid arthritis, osteoarthritis and multiple sclerosis. The immune system is weakened, leaving the body open to attack by infection and viral illnesses. Allergies may also result and, in the worst-case scenario, the body may respond by producing cancer cells.

Stress and the digestive system

The digestive system, which is particularly at risk, may show signs of stomach upsets, ulcers, irritable bowel and colitis. These problems with the digestive system are an important link to understanding chronic pain and the role that diet and nutrition play in making it worse, as well as in bringing about healing (see p. 54).

Stress is one of the major causes of the body's inability to digest food properly. It affects the acid levels in the stomach and interferes with the production of digestive enzymes. The whole system may become inflamed. As a result, if food is not digested properly, vitamins and minerals present in food cannot be utilized effectively to provide sufficient nutrition, which is important for repairing cells, growth, supporting teeth and bones, and maintaining a healthy blood supply – all factors that enable us to have sufficient energy to work and play and enjoy life generally. The digestion is further compromised as the raw materials needed to manufacture digestive enzymes are diminished, and we start a vicious circle of stress, poor digestion and increased stress, leading to even poorer digestion and, of course, exacerbation of any existing illnesses or chronic pain conditions.

Incorrectly digested food is a poisonous substance. It ferments and this produces toxicity. Normally, after food leaves the stomach it continues to be digested as it progresses through the gut, from where the nutrients pass into the bloodstream in order to be carried to wherever the body requires them. The gut has an immune defence system that detects any substances likely to cause harm to the body. Where inadequate digestion takes place the gut is overwhelmed and the lining can be damaged. This damage can result from infection, toxins or lack of digestive enzymes; in addition, the friendly bacteria of the gut that are needed for successful digestion may be replaced by unfriendly bacteria or other micro-organisms such as candida. The situation may be made worse by the consumption of antibiotics, processed foods, additives, too much alcohol or a poor diet in general.

Non-steroidal anti-inflammatory drugs, along with aspirin and its derivatives, often prescribed for pain and inflammation, can actually inflame the gut lining and become a problem in themselves. When the gut becomes inflamed or damaged, then improperly digested food and toxins, along with bacteria, viruses and yeasts may leak into the bloodstream and vital nutrients are lost because they are not absorbed. As a result, the lymphatic system and the liver, whose job is to deal with toxicity, become overworked and cannot cope and cease to function properly. They are under stress. When the gut is damaged in this way, the immune system becomes extremely sensitive and may mistake incorrectly digested food as an invader, giving rise to allergies.

Chronic pain results in unrelieved stress

We have seen that continued stress soon exhausts the body's ability to cope. People with pain may experience anxiety, depression and sleeplessness along with an increase in muscular tension and therefore further pain. They may develop digestive symptoms, especially if they are regularly taking medication. Anyone who shows signs of digestive distress in the form of bloating, heartburn, excessive wind, constipation, diarrhoea, stomach cramps or general bowel discomfort needs to address these problems, preferably by dealing with the toxicity and adjusting their diet. These symptoms are an indication that there may be food sensitivities, and the foods causing the problems should be investigated and excluded.

Those under severe prolonged stress may develop a weakened immune system and as a result lose the ability to ward off infections and other diseases, leaving them more susceptible to everything from colds and flu to cancer. In the 1960s, two American navy doctors, Thomas Holmes and Richard Rahe, carried out research on stress and its relationship to the ability of crew members to sustain long sea trips. They reported that someone who has experienced the death of a partner or a close family member, divorce, financial problems, birth of a new baby or moving home is more likely to experience serious illness within the next year. As this was one of my main areas of interest as a university teacher and when working on a project with families experiencing stress, I had some correspondence with these researchers, who provided me with some interesting background information to their study.

Another result of stress is that the arteries may become clogged by fats. Cholesterol is released into the blood vessels during the attempt to fight stress, and this may result in heart attack or stroke. These are probably the most extreme ways in which the body reacts to stress. There are many other disorders that may be manifested – headaches, insomnia, anxiety, depression and fatigue; and stress may be the basis for a number of chronic conditions.

10

Dealing with inflammation, water retention, sleeplessness

One of the problems that I faced when I first developed my chronic pain problem was presented by the fact that I could not be prescribed any form of aspirin, other anti-inflammatory drugs or corticosteroids because of the danger of stomach bleeding. I had to find other ways of coping because there did not seem to be a medical solution to the problem and the accompanying sleeplessness, weight gain and water retention – problems shared by many chronic pain sufferers. Fortunately my quest to find nutritional ways of dealing with my pain has also alleviated these other problems, as one might expect.

Inflammation is a response of the immune system to an injury or infection; it indicates that the body is dealing with the problem. It is also a characteristic of inflammatory illness such as arthritis. It produces heat, redness, pain, swelling and soreness. In the case of infection or injury, once the problem has been resolved, the inflammation usually dies down. However, in the case of an inflammatory illness, the body faces a constant battle to cope with inflammation; medically this is usually controlled by drugs.

Some people who have allergies and food sensitivities also experience inflammation in various parts of the body. In this case, inflammation may be seen as a pathological chemical reaction to a substance that is normally completely acceptable. In the case of allergy, the reaction can be instantaneous and the resulting inflammation and swellings can cause breathing difficulties, asthma attacks, choking, and irritation of the mucous membranes, the digestive tract and the bowel. The swellings may progress through the body or settle around the joints.

What happens when you have inflammation?

Inflammation is normally triggered by hormones and hormone-like substances such as prostaglandin E2, which are produced in the body as a defence when there is infection or injury present. It shows that there is increased blood flow and that the immune system is working well. Normally the hormones are switched off as soon as the inflammation has done its defensive job. In the case of inflammatory illness, or in food sensitivity, the hormones are out of balance. They continue to be produced when they are not needed, and inflammation becomes a problem. This imbalance is aggravated and inflammation increases if the diet is saturated with animal fats such as those found in red meat and dairy products and with the oils found in margarine, sunflower oil, corn oil, sesame oil and lard. These oils and fats stimulate the production of the inflammatory hormones to a level where they begin to attack the body, paving the way for the likelihood of further illness and disease.

In the case of food sensitivities, where the progression of the inflammatory response is not so rapid or exaggerated, the inflammation and swelling in the digestive tract can progressively limit the ability of the digestive system to absorb food completely. If a person is unaware that he or she has an allergy or food sensitivity then continued use of that food will further compromise the digestive tract and, what is more, build up even more inflammation around the joints, exacerbating pain problems.

Many health problems are inflammatory, which means that part of the body – such as a muscle or a joint, the gut or the respiratory tract – is inflamed. It is a sign that the body is reacting or over-reacting to something. There is little point in calming down an inflammation if the cause remains. The cause may be a food sensitivity, an inappropriate diet or another irritating substance such as alcohol.

The medical solution

Treating arthritis and other chronic pain conditions with pain-killers and anti-inflammatory drugs may be fine for a quick fix. However, while they dull down the pain they do nothing to remedy the underlying problems. In fact they may cause problems of their own, harming the liver, kidneys and digestive tract by increasing toxicity, thereby making the original problem worse. The most commonly used anti-inflammatory drugs are aspirin and ibuprofen. Paracetamol may be recommended for pain but it has little anti-inflammatory effect. Aspirin and ibuprofen fall within the general category of non-steroidal anti-inflammatory drugs. They do not sedate the person or depress the respiratory system. They are thought of as relatively safe.

There are problems, however, in that aspirin and ibuprofen can also adversely affect the digestive system, posing the risk of stomach bleeding and ulcer perforation, which can of course be extremely dangerous. I know this to my cost! In the 1950s, before people were aware that anyone could be allergic to these drugs, my life was threatened as a result of stomach bleeding after being prescribed aspirin for flu. It is estimated that up to 20 per cent of people experience indigestion as a result of using these drugs. Not only do they suffer irritation of the digestive tract but they can also suffer salt and fluid retention and renal impairment. There is even a risk of renal failure.

The dietary solution – the answer is in your food

There are many ways to reduce pain and inflammation without drugs. My book *Coping Successfully with Pain* demonstrated the use of exercise, relaxation and lifestyle changes, for example. Particularly important in these lifestyle changes is a diet rich in oily fish such as salmon, herring, sardines and mackerel, and in oils such as walnut, flax and hemp. These help the body produce different anti-inflammatory compounds such as prostaglandin E1 and prostaglandin E3.

And now – for my own special secret remedy which I would like to share with you – arrowroot.

Arrowroot

You are most likely to find arrowroot in the home-baking section of your local supermarket, but if not you can buy it at any health-food shop. It is derived from a plant, the maranta, found in various parts of the world including the West Indies, Central America, India, the Philippines and west Africa. It has been used since Roman times, generally as a food for invalids and babies and to alleviate the symptoms of stomach upset and bowel problems. I can remember my grandmother using it as a remedy for upset stomachs. By itself it has no taste. You may know it best as a thickener for soups, stews or fruit dishes. It is made up in the proportion of a tablespoon to 500 ml (1 pint) of water or milk, and it is prepared by taking a little of the cold liquid and making it into a smooth paste. Then the remainder of the liquid is boiled and, when boiling, added to the paste. The liquid is stirred well and it thickens up. If you wish you can add a little honey, cocoa or a flavouring of your choice. It can be eaten with stewed fruit or as a custard.

As far as I know, arrowroot has not been tested medically as an anti-inflammatory and I suppose it is not likely to be tested in this way while a lot of money is to be made from prescribing and selling anti-inflammatory drugs. It is my first line of defence against inflammation and I can take it knowing that it soon reduces internal swelling and leads quickly to eliminating excessive water.

My intolerance of wheat and milk causes the lining to be stripped away from my digestive system from the oesophagus through to the colon. I cannot prevent accidentally ingesting anything to which I am intolerant, and if I do I turn immediately to arrowroot, which gives my system protection, cutting out the likelihood of pain and discomfort. I have found that the symptoms that accompany wheat or dairy intake – bloating, cramps, weakness, and constipation or diarrhoea – are greatly reduced or do not occur at all if I am able to take arrowroot early enough. Because it is not a drug, arrowroot causes none of the nasty side-effects that often accompany drugs.

Water retention

Water retention develops over a long time. It is said that the body can retain 5 litres without it being apparent. It is a sure indication that the system has become toxic. If left untreated the toxicity can have a severe effect on the way the body functions. Often the first sign that I am retaining water is that I get a pressure headache or my ankles swell. I get unusually cold even when I am in a warm place, or I can sweat profusely without warning. It may take some time before I notice that my abdomen is distended and I have gained half a stone in weight. I know that when this stage is reached I am carrying a substantial amount of water. Apart from that, I have an increase in pain levels, I am unable to concentrate, I become lethargic and normal activities are suspended.

When you are retaining water there is a build-up of lactic acid in the body, and its toxicity causes pain and damage to the deep muscle tissues. There is no single magical solution to this problem. However, arrowroot will help the process of elimination, calcium can help to reduce the lactic acid levels, and magnesium will work towards ensuring more adequate sleep and reducing pain. Therefore it is advised that calcium and magnesium are always taken together because these two minerals assist each other in their work. Vitamin C not only aids the process of elimination but it also ensures the levels of the vitamin are maintained while so much water is being lost. To reduce the stress on your body further at such times it is a good idea to take a multivitamin and mineral supplement. This will prevent infection. Drinking plenty of water will flush out the salt, toxins, allergens and chemical stresses from your body. You can help further by cleansing the liver with milk thistle, also known as sylmarin, a herbal remedy obtainable from health-food shops in tablet form. I also find that onions and green vegetables, especially broccoli are a great help not only in removing excess water but also rebuilding damaged body tissues.

Anyone who is overweight is likely to be rewarded by tackling the problem of inflammation and water retention. The two go together like love and marriage. If you are working on removing toxicity then beware of releasing too many toxins too quickly into your liver, the cleansing organ of your body. Too many toxins released at once can give you headaches and flu-like symptoms, so remember to keep drinking plenty of water. Eating rice and grains is good for helping limit the effects of toxic release. Above all, maintain a diet in which vegetables, fruit, grains and seeds predominate and try to exclude, or at least to limit, animal fats, milk and other dairy produce, and saturated vegetable oils.

Sleeplessness

One of the major effects of chronic pain is the problem of insomnia, waking up in the middle of the night, or having difficulty in getting off to sleep. I recommend that you read the chapter on sleeplessness in my book *Coping Successfully with Pain*. Chronic pain not only produces disturbed sleep patterns but increases stress, anxiety and depression, which in turn affect your pain and your sleep. Inadequate nutrition and digestive problems also have an impact on sleep. In addition to following the advice already given about avoiding all those foods and drinks that add to chronic pain, you also need to avoid stimulants such as tea, coffee and alcoholic nightcaps. If you cannot avoid tea and coffee during the day then at least do not have any after sundown. You might have faith that the alcoholic nightcap helps to get you off to sleep but in fact it may be instrumental in causing you to wake up in the night. Do not have your evening meal later than 6.00 p.m. and avoid late snacks, which are difficult to digest. Cheese at bedtime is asking for trouble! Milky, sugary drinks at night can have a bad effect. The sugar may contribute to a lowering of blood sugar because it has the effect of raising the blood-sugar level very quickly and then just as quickly the blood-sugar levels drop suddenly. It is this sudden drop that brings about sleeplessness.

Milk is of course one of the trigger foods that may stimulate your pain. It also causes a lot of mucus to be produced, and this can affect your breathing and may induce snoring and wheeziness, which can disturb your sleep. You might find that valerian will help your body to relax and enable you to sleep more soundly. A cup of valerian, camomile or redbush tea at bedtime will have a tranquillizing effect. Include seeds, nuts, root and green leafy vegetables in your diet, since these are high in calcium and magnesium. These have a calming effect on your system.

Are supplements a good idea?

Inflammation, water retention, sleeplessness, pain and stress are inextricably interlinked with good nutrition. Just as bad effects can be aggravated by too many high-fat and sugary foods, they can be removed by cutting such foods out of your diet and replacing them with a good balance of healing foods.

Most nutritionists who work in the field of chronic pain advise that you should supplement your diet while you are making changes to it so that your level of vitamins and minerals is not reduced. Until your new healthy diet takes over, you will need additional nutritional help. The whole question of dietary supplementation would fill another book. I can only give general guidance and suggest that if you have a chronic pain problem and inflammation you would be well advised to seek help from a professional nutritionist. It will be money well spent. I can, however, share with you the fact that twice a year for about 2–3 months I boost my immune system by using multi-vitamins and minerals, vitamin C with bioflavinoids, and a vitamin B compound as well as using flaxseed oil and fish oil, zinc, magnesium and calcium. These all work towards boosting my general health and controlling inflammation. L-Glutamine is particularly important in helping to calm inflammation in the digestive system.

Anyone who is over 50, with an ageing digestive system, and particularly people with a degenerative chronic illness such as multiple sclerosis or arthritis, in which the production of natural enzymes has become sluggish, will benefit from taking digestive enzymes. These enzymes help to digest protein, carbohydrates and fats, and as a result partially digested food will not ferment in your system and cause additional absorption problems. Digestive enzymes can be readily obtained from health-food stores. You will need to seek guidance from a nutritionist if you think supplements will help you.

Buying supplements can be an expensive business but it is a good investment. However, you will be wasting your money if you rely solely on supplements and neglect to exercise, learn relaxation skills and make the essential dietary changes. If money is an issue then spend it on fruit and vegetables rather than supplements.

11

Recipes to get you started

One of the problems for people who have to be careful of their diet is that they can feel a burden to others, and there is a possibility that the pain sufferer will continue to eat the wrong things rather than upset the applecart. As a result the person may feel constantly unwell. It is important for everyone in the family to co-operate in finding a diet that suits everyone in the family and agree that healthy eating is the order of the day.

When preparing meals the golden rule should be fresh, preferably organic, ingredients, eaten raw or simply cooked using the herbs and spices recommended for their healing and cooling qualities. Salt must be used sparingly; instead, use a mixture of ground herbs for seasoning. If you have been accustomed to liberal amounts of salt and pepper in your food, the new flavours may seem strange at first but in time you will not need to have condiments on the table at all. The recipes here have been kept as simple as possible because I am well aware that standing for long periods preparing food is not the best thing for anyone with a pain problem.

The recipes have been selected from the many that my wife Eve has devised and adapted over the past 15 years. Some old favourites are naturally dairy- and gluten-free and involve none of the trigger foods. The dishes are first and foremost nutritious in that they provide all the vitamins and minerals necessary in a healthy diet. Because animal fats are avoided, the dishes ought to help anyone with a natural tendency to obesity problems, which often go with chronic illnesses and reduced mobility. The dishes also ought to go some way to repairing damage to the digestive system and rebalancing the metabolic processes in the body. Many people have gut damage resulting from the stress of their illness, from eating the wrong foods such as red meat and animal fats, or from eating too much and too quickly. With a diet such as this it should not be necessary to resort to antacids or other digestive tablets.

The dishes are designed to make few demands on the digestive system, so many of the recipes suggest chopping or slicing food finely and it is recommended that you eat smaller meals more often. Do not try to keep up with those who do not feel satisfied until they have to loosen their belts! By eating to the limit, food passes through the gut undigested, thus exacerbating poor absorption and poor nutrition, which of course can lead to further stress and an increase in pain.

Suggested ingredients for your store cupboard

All good home cooking starts by having the ingredients readily to hand.

The ingredients listed here are ones that you can keep by you to get you started on a diet that eliminates wheat or gluten and dairy products, because these are the major triggers. As you become more attuned to your new eating habits you will be able to extend the list:

- almonds and walnuts (plain, unsalted);
- arrowroot for thickening (you can find this in the bakery section of your supermarket);
- black peppercorns;
- bread and bread mixes – you must not expect gluten-free bread to taste like normal wheat bread: it is the gluten in wheat that gives that springy feel to a loaf. Gluten-free bread is available in supermarkets and I find it quite acceptable as a substitute but it is rather crumbly in texture and it needs to be heated in the microwave or toasted to make it palatable. Gluten-free bread enables you to enjoy toast with toppings – beans on gluten-free crackers doesn't really work! There are some quite good bread mixes on the market, which just need water or oil adding before cooking. You will have to experiment with these to find the one you prefer. Most seem to come from Australia, a country that is leading the gluten-free products market;
- eggs (if you can tolerate them);
- flours – brown rice flour (unprocessed), gram flour (chickpea); buckwheat (which does not belong to the wheat family), potato flour;
- cooking oil – olive oil, walnut oil, hemp oil;
- cornflakes (gluten-free) or muesli (gluten-free);
- dried fruit (sulphur- and additive-free);
- tinned fish – particularly tuna, sardines, salmon;
- fruit or vegetable drinks and purées (except citrus fruits);
- polenta;
- pulses – dried red lentils or green lentils, tins of chickpeas, red kidney beans, baked beans (check that they are gluten-free);
- sea salt;

- soya products as substitutes for dairy products – soya milk, soya desserts, soya ice-cream – provided that you are not sensitive to soya. Braised tofu (tinned) is a most useful standby – made from soya, it can be used hot or cold and is delicious used in place of bacon with a fried egg for breakfast. (Braised tofu is my three-year-old grandson's favourite food!);
- sugar (but you are aiming at reducing this drastically – remember that cooked dates or date syrup make a healthier substitute for cane sugar, as do pear and apple concentrate and agave syrup); avoid chemical sweeteners;
- tea or coffee (if you can tolerate them), but better for you are green tea, rooibos (redbush tea) and herbal teas, and these teas are good if you are milk-intolerant since they are pleasant to drink without any addition.

We sometimes use some of the foods that may be responsible for triggering pain. When you embark on the process of eliminating trigger foods from your diet, you will need either to leave out the whole recipe or exclude that ingredient from the recipe. Once you have established which of these foods are triggers for your pain, then these must be left out of your diet permanently. Build your diet based on the safe foods. A note of caution, however. Even if you have found some of the foods in the list of trigger foods to be safe, then I would recommend that you eat these in moderation. You may be able to get away with eating small amounts infrequently but we are not always aware of the cumulative adverse effects that are building up in our system until difficulties arise. As you will see, very few, if any, of the recipes contain refined sugar – many recipe books that concentrate on healthy eating still use sugar freely and it is difficult to understand why. In preparing these recipes, Eve has tried to find healthy alternatives to sugar, and I am sure that you will find her suggestions nutritionally very useful.

Common healing ingredients

The recipes are accompanied by comments about the nutritional value and healing quality of many of the ingredients especially when being used for the first time. However, three of the ingredients are basic to many of the recipes – onions, olive oil and ginger.

Onions

Onions, shallots, spring onions, leeks and chives are from the same family and are used almost universally to provide flavour to most savoury cooking. I only have to smell an onion cooking to have my taste buds stimulated. They are rich in vitamins A, B and C and in minerals – magnesium, phosphorus, potassium and essential natural sulphur compounds. They are also rich in bioflavinoids, which help the assimilation of vitamin C. Bioflavinoids occur naturally in many foods, such as citrus fruits, green vegetables and onions. They are a complex group of substances that have an antioxidant action that helps to improve vascular health and prevent heart disease by reducing levels of blood cholesterol and preventing blood clots.

Onions are a valuable food for anyone with arthritis, rheumatic pain or period pain because they ease fluid retention and promote the elimination of urea, a chemical produced by the body as part of the waste disposal system. A build-up of urea can make inflammatory conditions worse.

Olive oil

Olive oil is probably not always the best oil for culinary purposes as it can be a little heavy. However, it is ideal when you want to combine its nutritional and medicinal qualities with your diet. Olives and olive oil form the basis of the diet in the Mediterranean area, where the use of animal fats in cooking is minimal compared with northern Europe. In the countries where olive oil is used widely there is a low incidence of cardiovascular disease. Olives contain the vitamins A and E and the minerals phosphorus, potassium and manganese, as well as antioxidants. Perhaps more importantly its oil is useful in maintaining a balance in the cholesterol levels in the blood and preventing fatty deposits being laid down in the arteries, and as a consequence reducing heart disease, blood clots and strokes. Anyone with chronic pain needs to have a good blood flow to all parts of the body and this is where olive oil plays its part.

We prefer to use extra virgin olive oil obtained from the first cold pressing of the olives. It is this first cold pressing that draws out all the nutritional benefits from the olives. It is well worth the little extra cost to buy the best, especially if you are giving up deep frying as a means of cooking and avoiding saturated animal fats. Do not be tempted to buy cheap refined olive oil. When you buy this it is like buying any other processed food where most of the benefits have been lost in the treatment. Extra virgin olive oil when combined with lemon juice or wine vinegar and herbs makes the perfect salad dressing. Medicinally, it can be taken by mouth either by itself or mixed with a little lemon juice each morning before breakfast. It is very helpful in easing the ravages of stress and poor food absorption in the digestive system. It is often recommended as a remedy for constipation which can result from the use of prescription medicines.

Recently Eve and I were talking to the owner of a music shop in Spain who gave us his recipe for a healthy life. First thing each morning he ate a clove of raw garlic and followed this with a tablespoon of good olive oil, which he claimed prevented any unpleasant smell on his breath. He kept a bag of almonds in his pockets which he snacked on throughout the day. (If you want to try this at home be careful of your teeth!) He maintained that these three ingredients kept him in peak condition, and his appearance gave us every reason to believe him. Olives can be made into pesto or tapenade, which can be used as toppings or spreads. Pesto and tapenade can be made at home or bought from good grocers. Many ready-made brands of pesto include cheese, so read the label to check.

Ginger

Ginger blocks histamine and also inhibits prostaglandins, chemicals that trigger inflammation. Studies suggest that people who have migraines can be helped by taking ½ to 1 teaspoon of ground ginger each day. I take ginger in this way from time to time for short periods because I believe it helps to combat the inflammation, swelling and joint stiffness that lies at the root of my pain. Because I cannot take prescribed drugs, I am always on the lookout for ways to control inflammation. You cannot overdose on ginger and it has only beneficial effects. You do not need to take it all at once on a spoon – you can sprinkle it on food, use it in cooking or even add it to your marmalade. It is worth trying ginger over a period of three months before making a judgement about its usefulness for you. There are also many ginger teas on the market.

Since digestive problems seem to accompany many of the common pain disorders, it is worth using ginger as a digestive aid. It does not matter whether you take powdered ginger or grated root ginger – both work in exactly the same way. Besides having anti-inflammatory effects, ginger reduces nausea and has a calming effect on the stomach and bowel, thus promoting healing. It is possible to buy ginger in capsule form as a food supplement if you do not fancy the taste.

Garlic

Many things have been claimed for garlic as a healing agent or for prevention of health problems. It is part of the onion family and has been used for thousands of years as a health-giving food. It was used in ancient times to promote strength, increase resistance to infection and ward off the plague, and during the nineteenth century it was used widely to ward off cholera during the many epidemics. Its active ingredient is an oil called allicin, which can break down blood clots. It promotes good circulation and helps to reduce blood pressure. It encourages cholesterol to be eliminated from the blood vessels. It is known to work against bacterial and fungal complaints. Like ginger, it is a useful digestive aid and helps to restore the balance of bacteria in the system. It is known to boost the immune system. It works best when eaten raw. However, it is possible to obtain odourless garlic capsules. In addition, olive oil can be used to combat the bad breath that garlic can cause, as can caraway seeds, cardamom seeds and parsley leaves. Some cooks use a sprig of parsley in conjunction with garlic in their cooking.

Some cooking hints

Traditionalists would say that soup stock should be made from scratch, and certainly this is a good way to use up vegetable parings and scraps of meat, and it does make all the difference to the taste of soups. However, taking into account the time taken in preparing a meal, I think it is quite in order to use stock cubes – but make sure that they do not contain ingredients that may not agree with you, and remember that they contain a lot of salt, so you will not need to add extra salt to your cooking. There are some very good vegan and gluten-free powdered gravies and sauces available at good-quality supermarkets or your local health-food shop. The same goes for seasonings, and if you are using soy sauce make sure you get the wheat-free variety.

A number of the recipes in this book stem from the time when I found it impossible to stand for longer than it took to peel four potatoes, and this is probably the experience of many people with chronic pain.

'Sweat' the vegetables rather than frying or sautéing them, because oil starts to become toxic at higher temperatures. 'Sweating' means that you place the vegetables in oil at a low temperature and slowly cook them, uncovered, stirring with a wooden spoon until they are cooked through. This can take about 20 minutes depending on the type of vegetable used. If this is not a problem then this is a good way to get the full benefit from the vegetables. If you have health problems then make it a rule never to cook in hot oil.

Steam-fried vegetables

Steam frying is even better for you. Do exactly as you would when using oil but use water instead. Choose from the following vegetables: potatoes, sweet potatoes, parsnips, carrots, squashes, courgettes, broccoli or cauliflower florets. Add strips of chicken, duck or turkey. Start by heating up your wok or saucepan and add a very small amount of water (about 2 or 3 tablespoons). It will sizzle in the pan. Then add chopped onion, chopped or crushed garlic, finely chopped root ginger or 1 teaspoon of ground ginger, cumin or coriander powder or seeds and keep turning them over in the water. When the pan looks dry add another couple of tablespoons of hot water and keep turning until the onion is transparent. Then add the root vegetables, cut into small pieces, and thin strips of chicken, duck or turkey. Keep adding small amounts of hot water as required and turning the food so that all parts have contact with the hot pan. After 5 minutes add the florets. Seasoning can be added to taste. I prefer to use a dash of tamari soy sauce or mixed herbs instead of the usual salt and pepper.

You can make a sweet and sour sauce to give additional flavour by mixing together a small amount of olive oil with apricot conserve or marmalade and a dash of lemon juice.

For a hotter dish you can add a small amount of chilli flakes, but do not use too much. Add it in pinches rather than spoonfuls!

I found this method of cooking ideal when my standing time was limited because of pain.

Steaming

From experience I find it better to steam vegetables in the microwave or to use a Chinese wooden steamer over a pan of hot water and then finish the vegetables in a hot wok for 2–3 minutes in a few tablespoons of hot water to which you have already added herbs and spices. You can always drizzle cold olive oil over the vegetables as a glaze just before serving.

All of these methods of cooking ensure the maximum nutritional benefit from your food. Because little or no fat is used you will not put on weight unless you overeat.

Soups and starters

Most of these soup recipes use grains, pulses and vegetables as their base; where meat is used it is poultry rather than red meat and it is finely sliced or chopped. Thickening is provided by arrowroot or potato flour and no dairy products are included. When making soups you can always make more than you need and freeze the surplus in plastic containers.

Vegetable soup
Serves 3–4

Ingredients

1 medium-sized onion, peeled and sliced
1 garlic clove (optional)
1 tbsp olive oil
1 small turnip, peeled and sliced
500 ml (1 pint) water

1 small parsnip, if liked, peeled and sliced
1 medium potato, peeled and sliced
4 or 5 broccoli florets

tamari-type gluten-free sauce (you may have to get this from a health-food shop)

Method

1 Fry the onion (and garlic if using) in the oil on medium heat.
2 Add the vegetables and about half of the water. Bring to boil, cover and simmer for about 20 minutes.
3 Add the remainder of the water to cool the vegetables down before liquidizing them. If you do not have a liquidizer use a potato masher to break down the vegetables.
4 Return soup to the pan and heat through again, adding the tamari sauce and further seasoning to taste. You should not require any additional salt as the tamari sauce tastes quite salty.
5 If you like a slightly thicker soup add a paste of 1 tsp arrowroot or potato flour stirred into a small amount of water.

If liked, you can add 1 tbsp chopped parsley just before serving. For a quick version of this recipe use a pack of frozen mixed vegetables.

Lentil soup
Serves 3–4

Ingredients

250 g dried lentils
1 large onion, peeled and sliced
1 garlic clove (crushed)
1 tbsp vegetable oil
2.5 cm (1 inch) root ginger or
   ½ tsp ground ginger

500 ml (1 pint) boiling water
1 tbsp tamari-type gluten-free
   sauce
250 g carrots, washed, trimmed
   and sliced
½ red pepper, diced

ground mixed herbs for flavouring (I find that Herbemare™ is a good mixture of herbs that contains a minimal amount of salt)

Method

1 Pick over the lentils for small stones, then put them in a large bowl and wash them under the tap and drain in a mesh sieve.
2 In a large saucepan put the oil, onion, garlic and ginger and fry for 3–4 minutes.
3 Add the lentils and stir into the onion mix. Cook for 1 minute.
4 Pour in the boiling water and tamari sauce.
5 Add carrots and peppers.
6 Bring back to the boil, cover and simmer for 25 minutes. If the soup becomes too thick, add more boiling water.
7 Season to taste.

Cream of leek soup
Serves 3–4

This soup is very gentle on the digestive system and, while it is very tasty, it also clears away toxicity.

Ingredients

1 tbsp olive oil
2 medium leeks, thoroughly
   washed and finely chopped
¼ cup brown rice

500 ml (1 pint) boiling water
500 ml (1 pint) chicken stock or
   gluten-free bouillon

Method

1 Take a large saucepan and pour in enough boiling water to cover the bottom.

2 Add the rice with the leeks and cook for 1 minute.
3 Add the remainder of water and stock, and cook until the rice is tender.
4 Season to taste and allow to cool. Add the oil at this point.
5 When cool, purée in a blender or use a potato masher to achieve a purée consistency.
6 Reheat, adjust seasoning to taste and serve.

Broccoli and leek soup
Serves 3–4

This soup helps to relieve water retention and inflammation from the digestive system and is very easily digested.

Ingredients

1 tbsp olive oil
½ large onion, finely chopped
2 medium leeks, finely chopped
4 or 5 broccoli florets
500 ml (1 pint) water

¼ tsp ground ginger
¼ tsp ground coriander
fresh coriander, fresh basil
  (optional)
seasoning

As an optional extra you can sprinkle each bowl with a little dairy-free/gluten-free 'parmesan cheese' substitute, available at some supermarkets in their 'free from' section. If available, a couple of sprigs of fresh coriander or basil can be used to top off each bowl.

Method

1 Heat the oil in a medium saucepan.
2 Add the onion, ginger and coriander and cook until the onion is transparent.
3 Add the leeks with half the water.
4 Bring to the boil, cover and simmer for 5 minutes.
5 Add broccoli florets and simmer, covered, for 10–15 minutes.
6 Season and allow to cool. When cool, blend ingredients together in liquidizer or mash the vegetables to form a purée.
7 Reheat, and just before serving sprinkle the top with a little dairy-free and gluten-free 'parmesan cheese'. Adjust seasoning as necessary.

Easy tomato soup
Serves 3–4

Although tomatoes are listed among the trigger foods, they are a very nutritious food for anyone who is not adversely affected by them. They contain vitamins A, B and C, folic acid, minerals and antioxidants. They are helpful for the digestive system as they reduce inflammation. They help to prevent the formation of uric acid crystals, are good for bones and joints, and help to relieve rheumatoid arthritis and rheumatism. Use organic tomatoes where possible.

I learned this recipe when watching a cookery programme on Spanish television. I hope I understood what the chef was saying! However, we have made this several times and it is most enjoyable. It can also be used as a pasta sauce by limiting the boiling water to no more than ½ cup.

Ingredients

½ cup olive oil
1 400 g (14 oz) tin chopped
  tomatoes
2 tsp paprika or ground pimento
1 medium onion
1 bay-leaf

2 tbsp ground almonds
½ tsp turmeric
2.5 cm (1 inch) root ginger, cut
  into thin strips
750 ml (1½ pints) boiling water
scant ½ tsp sea salt

Method

1 Heat half the oil in a heavy-bottomed saucepan.
2 Add the onions, garlic, turmeric and ginger and the paprika or pimento, and cook until the onions are soft.
3 Add the ground almonds and continue stirring for a further 2 minutes. Do not worry if it looks quite dry at this stage.
4 Add the remainder of the oil and continue to stir in well.
5 Add the tin of chopped tomatoes, salt, water and bay-leaf. Stir thoroughly and allow to simmer for 15 minutes. Adjust seasoning as necessary before serving.

Pumpkin and carrot soup
Serves 3–4

Pumpkins make a lovely soup because they break down to form a smooth textured purée of a rich orange colour and subtle flavour. Pumpkins are known to be calming and cooling and therefore they are often advised for people who suffer from insomnia. They are easy on the digestive system. Carrots are a rich source of antioxidants. They are recommended because they boost the immune system and help to reduce cholesterol in the blood; they are rich in minerals and beta-carotene, which the body converts into vitamin A. Carrots can be eaten on a daily basis to advantage, raw as crudités, grated in salad, as a cooked vegetable, soup, or as a healthy drink.

Ingredients

1 large onion
1 tsp ground cinnamon
450 g (1 lb) pumpkin flesh
2 large carrots
3.5 cm (1½ inches) fresh ginger, grated

1 bay-leaf
black pepper
600 ml (20 fl oz) vegetable stock
600 ml (20 fl oz) hot water

Method

1 Dice the onion and place in a saucepan with 2 tbsp boiling water. Set heat to medium and cook the onion until it is soft.
2 Wash the pumpkin and dice the flesh into small pieces (you do not need to remove the skin unless it is marked or rough), and slice the carrots.
3 Add the pumpkin and carrots to the pan and continue to cook until the vegetables begin to soften.
4 Add the grated ginger to the pan along with the stock, water, cinnamon and bay-leaf. Bring to the boil and simmer until all the vegetables are tender. Remove the bay-leaf.
5 Using a potato masher, mash the vegetables until the pumpkin breaks up. Season to taste.

If you wish you can sprinkle with a little grated orange peel before serving.

Spring onion, garlic and clove soup
Serves 3–4

This soup has a number of healing effects. It is very calming to the digestive system and will ease water retention because of its anti-inflammatory effects. Besides the other ingredients already discussed above, it contains cloves, which have an anaesthetic effect (as many of you will know since they can soothe toothache). In addition, cloves can combat intestinal infections. This soup is very low in calories and contains no fat whatsoever so is very useful for anyone wishing to control their weight. If you have a cold it will help bring down your temperature and ease the unpleasant symptoms. It might be said to be a vegetable 'hot toddy'.

Ingredients

6–10 spring onions
3 garlic cloves, crushed
1 tsp ground ginger or about
   5 cm (2 inches) ginger root,
   grated

2 cloves
2 tbsp chopped celery
1 litre (2 pints) water
seasoning to taste

Method

Boil all ingredients together for 15 minutes and serve hot.
As a variation, cubes of firm tofu can be added to the recipe near the end.

Carrot and coriander soup
Serves 3–4

Coriander blends well with carrots. It is known to have beneficial effects on the digestion, and it is helpful to anyone who has irritable bowel syndrome or is experiencing problems as a result of taking prescription drugs for pain or inflammation. It contains vitamin B and folic acid. The seeds are much more useful than the leaves as far as medicinal qualities are concerned. Both the leaves and the seeds can be sprinkled over salads or soups.

Ingredients

1 small onion
225 g (8 oz) carrots, washed and
   peeled
1 tsp ground coriander or
   coriander seeds
1 tbsp olive oil

few fresh coriander leaves for
   garnish
boiling water sufficient to cover
   the carrots
salt and pepper to taste

Method

1 Chop the onion and steam fry in a small amount of boiling water until transparent.
2 Slice the carrots into 2.5 cm (1 inch) pieces and add to the onion along with the water, olive oil and seasoning. Simmer until the carrots are just cooked.
3 Allow to cool slightly then put into a blender or food processor and purée.
4 Reheat and adjust seasoning.
5 Before serving sprinkle with chopped fresh coriander leaves.

Nev's winter warmer
Serves 2

This soup is also delicious used as a pasta sauce or served cold as a summer soup. It is a good way of using up small amounts of vegetables or juices getting near their use-by date.

Ingredients

5–7.5 cm (2–3 inches) sweet potato, chopped
2.5 cm (1 inch) ginger, grated or finely sliced, or ½ tsp ground ginger
1 tsp cinnamon
½ red pepper

5 cm (2 inches) cucumber, peeled and chopped
500 ml (1 pint) water
250 ml (½ pint) vegetable or tomato juice
pinch chilli flakes
½ tsp sea salt

Method

1 Place all ingredients except salt and chilli into medium saucepan with enough water to cover.
2 Bring to boil and simmer gently until the sweet potato is cooked through.
3 Then add sea salt and chilli flakes, and stir well. Allow to cool slightly and put through a food processor or blender.
4 Add more hot water as desired and mix well.
5 Serve with fingers of toast.

Main meals

Most of the main meals below are based on vegetables, pulses and grains, since virtually all nutrients can be obtained from these ingredients, and they are the least likely foods to cause problems for people with pain or food sensitivity. They place fewer demands than other foods on a sensitive digestive system. Anything containing animal fat has largely been excluded because of the problems of absorption and the bad effect that animal fats have on the arteries. However, if you cannot wean yourself from meat then you are free to add it to these recipes, but I would suggest you add only a small amount for its flavour and try to restrict it to poultry or rabbit because these meats are likely to cause fewer problems than other meats.

You will see that margarine is not used in any of the recipes, because it contains 'trans' fats, which have a bad effect on the arteries, impeding blood flow. Anyone experiencing pain needs a good flow of blood to all parts of the body, especially the painful areas.

Fish is often criticized because it does not contain much fibre, but fish such as salmon, mackerel, herring and tuna are rich in omega-3 oils and in vitamin D, which works together with calcium to help to strengthen bones. Fish recipes are included because some of you, like myself, may find that you feel so much better on a diet that is mainly vegetable but that includes fish. It is a good alternative to red meat and should be an essential part of the diet of anyone with an inflammatory illness because of its anti-inflammatory action. It is beneficial to anyone who suffers from multiple sclerosis, high blood pressure or ulcerative colitis. Anyone who has a water retention problem, which often accompanies arthritis, will be helped considerably by eating fish frequently. If fresh fish is not available then use canned, unboned sardines, mackerel, herring and tuna.

If you have no problem with wheat and milk you may, as a birthday treat, be forgiven for indulging in deep-fried battered fish! It is not to be recommended, particularly because the fat is used over and over again and becomes more toxic each time it is used, and because the fat may be animal fat.

The recipes below have been selected to appeal to the taste-buds and to the eye and to show that the diet described in this book can be just as enjoyable as any other – you will not feel in any way deprived.

Pasta with tomato sauce
Serves 3–4 (sauce)

Many commercially available pasta sauces are highly processed and may be bulked out with wheat and highly refined sugars. This recipe will give you a tasty sauce that can be used with pasta (gluten-free pastas are readily available), rice or quinoa, and any surplus can be frozen. Make it some time before it is needed because this sauce improves by standing for 30 minutes so that the flavours can blend.

Ingredients

2 tbsp extra-virgin olive oil
pinch fennel seeds
1 tsp dried basil
1 tsp dried oregano
1 tsp paprika or ground pimento
4 garlic cloves, crushed
½ tsp sea salt or tamari sauce, if required
1 bay-leaf
1 medium onion, finely chopped

1 small carrot, peeled and finely grated
1 tin Italian tomatoes, mashed (avoid any brands that contain anything other than tomatoes and citric acid – many cheaper varieties list various additives, including sugar, which is to be avoided)
1 carton passata

Method

1 Heat the olive oil over a medium heat, and into it put the basil, oregano, fennel seeds and paprika, along with the onion, carrot and garlic. Cook for 10 minutes. Do not allow to burn.
2 Add the crushed tomatoes and passata and continue cooking for another 20 minutes or until the desired thickness is reached. If you think it is getting too thick just add a little boiling water. Add salt or tamari sauce to taste, if necessary.
3 Rest the sauce for 30 minutes so that the ingredients can blend.

Patrick's Ardèche quinoa risotto
Serves 2

We met Patrick while caravanning in the Ardèche area of France. He was wearing the white jacket and chequer-board trousers associated with chefs. He spoke English with a strong French-cum-Welsh accent, which intrigued us. He explained that he had just returned from Thailand, where his contract had finished, and he was on our camp-site to help his brother, who ran the site restaurant. At one time he had been the resident chef at Theatre Clwyd in North Wales and had married a Welsh girl (hence the accent). He was keen for us to patronize the site restaurant and offered to cook any dish that we wanted. As a challenge we asked him what he could do with a packet of quinoa, which at that time was little known. Nutritionally, quinoa is superior to all other grains, though in fact it is not a grain but a seed. It is a complete protein as it contains all eight essential amino acids, a range of minerals – phosphorus, magnesium, iron and zinc, together with omega-3, -6 and -9 oils. It is naturally gluten-free. It was known as the 'food of the gods' by the ancient Incas. It can be used in stir-fries, soups, stews or salads and, when cooked with rice or soya milk, it can be made into a breakfast porridge to which you can add fruit, dried fruit or nuts. Because of its high protein content it makes a good substitute for meat. It is best prepared with other, stronger-flavoured ingredients because it takes on their flavours. It can be used as an alternative to rice or potatoes.

This is the dish that Patrick prepared for us.

Method for the quinoa

1 Take one measure of quinoa to two measures of boiling water – 70 g (2.5 oz) of quinoa is recommended for each person.
2 Mix the quinoa and water in a medium to large saucepan and cook for 10 minutes over a moderate heat.
3 Remove from heat, cover and leave so that quinoa can absorb the remaining water.

Ingredients for the risotto

1 tbsp olive oil
1 small onion
1 garlic clove
½ green pepper
½ red pepper

1 tbsp garden peas
2.5 cm (1 inch) root ginger, grated
Pinch chilli flakes
seasoning to taste

Method

1 Finely chop the onion, garlic and peppers.
2 In a large frying pan or wok, heat the olive oil over a moderate heat and stir in all the above ingredients except the peas. Stir for 5 minutes.
3 Add the peas and the cooked quinoa and heat through.

A variety of vegetables or tinned fish such as tuna or sardines can be used in this dish, which can be served hot or cold.

This is a good dish to prepare in advance because it will store in the fridge for a day or two.

Kedgeree
Serves 3

Making kedgeree is a good way to use up left-over cooked rice.

Although this is a traditional breakfast dish, kedgeree can be enjoyed at any time. Suitable fish include haddock, sea bream, turbot, hake, halibut, salmon and cod. If using smoked fish make sure it has not been chemically dyed. You can usually tell by the colour – naturally smoked fish is much paler in colour. If in doubt, check with your supplier.

Ingredients

1 tbsp olive oil
225 g (8 oz) cooked or cured fish
  (cold)
1 egg, hard-boiled

1 egg, well beaten
120 g (4 oz) cooked rice
salt and pepper to taste
parsley or basil to garnish

Method

1 Skin, bone and flake the fish.
2 Put olive oil into a medium saucepan. Stir in the fish, rice, pepper and salt, and the chopped-up white part only of the hard-boiled egg.
3 Add the beaten egg to the other ingredients. Stir over heat until very hot then place on serving dish.
4 Rub the yolk of the hard-boiled egg through a sieve over the fish. Garnish with parsley or basil.

Stir-fried rice with tofu
Serves 4

This is another way of using up left-over cooked rice.

Tofu is a very useful ingredient, and it is full of protein, vitamins and minerals. It is made from soya bean curd. It has no flavour of its own but will absorb flavour from other ingredients. A little tamari sauce beaten into tofu makes a simple sauce or dressing.

Ingredients

1 tbsp olive oil
1 small onion or 3 spring onions
  (scallions), chopped
1 garlic clove, peeled and finely
  chopped
1 tbsp fresh ginger root, peeled
  and grated

1 package (175 g, 6 oz) tofu, cubed
2 cups cooked rice
1 tbsp wheat-free soy sauce
½ cup tinned peas
1 tsp fresh coriander leaves,
  chopped, or ½ tsp dried
  coriander

Method

1 In a wok or large frying pan heat the olive oil and sauté the onion, garlic, ginger and dried coriander, if using. Stir constantly with a wooden spoon.
2 Add the cubed tofu and warm it through.
3 Add the cooked rice, stirring and turning to mix with the other ingredients, until warmed through.
4 Add the soy sauce (tamari if you are wheat-sensitive), the peas and the fresh coriander, if using, and mix well.

Mediterranean roasted vegetables

This dish can be made from a selection of any vegetables, but my preference is for red onions, carrots, swede, parsnips, aubergines, courgettes, celery and beef tomatoes.

Method

1 Wash, peel and cut onions and any other root vegetables you are using into 5 cm (2 inch) cubes or strips and lay them on the bottom of the dish. It is best to use the largest roasting dish or tin that will fit into your oven. That way the vegetables can be placed on the base of the dish in a single layer.
2 Sprinkle well with olive oil and place in a hot oven. Roast for 25–30 minutes, turning every 10 minutes. Do not allow the vegetables to burn.
3 In the mean time, wash, dry and cut any non-root vegetables, such as peppers, tomatoes, courgettes or aubergines, into cubes or strips. Add these to the roasting dish and sprinkle with a little more olive oil. If you wish you can add a whole bulb of garlic, having first of all cut 1 cm (½ inch) off the top (no need to peel). You can now also sprinkle in your favourite herbs if you wish – this is preferable to using salt.

4 Cook for a further 20–25 minutes until all the vegetables are tender. You will know when the dish is ready when the root vegetables can be pierced with a fork.

Nev's favourite fish dish
Serves 2

This dish allows you to choose your own favourite fish from a selection of mackerel, salmon, tuna, herring, trout, sea bass or red snapper. For convenience, the recipe here uses mackerel, which is rich in omega-3 oils, is full of flavour and, best of all, is much cheaper than sea bass or red snapper! It is served with a salsa verde.

If you have a problem with tomatoes, leave them out and serve on a bed of mixed salad leaves or roasted vegetables.

Ingredients for the tomatoes and fish

1 mackerel fillet per person
1 450 g (1 lb) tin chopped tomatoes in tomato juice containing no artificial additives

1 tbsp olive oil
1 garlic clove, chopped
1 tsp herbes de Provence
pinch sea salt

Method for the tomatoes and fish

1 Drain any liquid from the tomatoes and empty them into a wok or a deep-sided frying pan.
2 Stir in the olive oil, garlic, herbs and salt, and heat gently until all is hot.
3 While this is cooking, brush the fish fillets with oil and grill on both sides.
4 When the fish is cooked, remove it from the heat and place it on a warmed plate on a bed of tomato mixture. Before serving, pour over the salsa verde.

Ingredients for the salsa verde

Handful fresh basil leaves, finely chopped
1 tbsp olive oil

1 garlic clove, crushed
pinch sea salt

Method for the salsa verde

Add olive oil and garlic to the basil, and blend together with a pinch of sea salt.

Duck breast with red onion marmalade
Serves 2

Life is very dull if you do not give yourself treats, so here is one of my favourites – the recipe uses duck, the fat of which, in moderation, is easily tolerated.

Ingredients for the duck

1 duck breast
Mixed herbs
1 garlic clove, thinly sliced

Method for the duck

1 Wipe and dry the duck breast on kitchen paper, then make diagonal cuts an inch apart across the meaty side, cutting slightly into the fat.
2 Sprinkle the herbs into the cuts and insert the slices of garlic. Brush the lean side with a little oil to prevent it drying out.
3 Place the pan on a medium heat and lay the duck in the pan, skin side down. Gently cook with a lid on the pan for 10 minutes.
4 The aim is to let the duck cook in its own juices. Check that it does not dry out. If it seems to be drying out, add a couple of tablespoons of hot water. Test with a fork for tenderness. You may prefer to let it cook for a further 5 minutes. Leave to stand for a few minutes then finely slice at an angle. Serve with the onion marmalade and a small salad.

Ingredients for the marmalade

1 tbsp olive oil
2 red onions, peeled and sliced or cut into rings
1 tbsp date syrup

Method for the marmalade

1 Heat the olive oil and gently sweat the onions, making sure you do not allow them to burn.
2 When soft, turn up the heat, add the date syrup and cook for 5 minutes, stirring all the time until the mixture turns dark and takes on the consistency of marmalade.
3 Allow to cool slightly before serving.

Smoked salmon and prawn salad
Serves 2

This is a useful dish if you are in a hurry.

Ingredients

A few slices smoked salmon
5 or 6 large frozen prawns
lemon juice
1 cucumber

1 small carton plain soya
  yoghurt or mayonnaise
mixed salad leaves

Method

1 Thaw the prawns in the microwave.
2 Mix in a bowl with a sprinkling of lemon juice.
3 Chop the cucumber and mix with yoghurt or mayonnaise.
4 Place salad leaves on plate, lay smoked salmon on the leaves and arrange the prawns on top of it. To finish, spoon on the yoghurt or mayonnaise dressing.

Turkey mince curry with rice
Serves 2

This is not a hot curry. It uses a combination of spices. If you want a hotter flavour then add some chilli flakes or powder. If you wish, a few steamed vegetables can be served separately.

On no account use commercially produced curry powder as it may contain wheat.

Ingredients

225 g (8 oz) turkey mince
  (vegetarians can use soya
  mince)
1 garlic clove, crushed
2 tbsp vegetable oil
1 tsp ground cloves
1 tsp cumin seeds
1 tsp cinnamon
1 tsp grated ginger

1 tsp chopped fresh coriander, or
  flat parsley if you cannot find
  coriander
3 cardamom pods, bruised,
  or ¼ tsp ground cardamom
5 dried, sulphur-free apricots
  (these are a dark brown colour),
  chopped
1 cup hot vegetable stock or
  water

Method for the curry sauce

1 In a medium saucepan or wok, bring the oil to medium heat.
2 Into the heated oil, place the cumin seeds, garlic and cloves.
3 When the cumin seeds begin to darken, add the cinnamon, ginger and cardamom.
4 Stir together for 30 seconds, then add the turkey mince and chopped apricots, and stir thoroughly.
5 Add the stock or water, bring back to a bubbling boil, and then turn down the heat to simmering point. Cook for a further 5 minutes, checking that the sauce does not dry out.
6 Check for taste and add a little sea salt or herb salt if necessary, but I find that it does not require additional salt if you use a stock.
7 Turn off the heat and leave for 30 minutes so that the flavours can blend.
8 When the rice is cooked you can return the sauce to the heat for a couple of minutes to reheat it.

Ingredients for the rice

Brown basmati rice (1 cup dry rice will serve 2)
½ tbsp vegetable oil

2 cups boiling water to each cup of rice
½ tsp sea salt

Method for the rice

1 Wash the rice in a large bowl, rubbing the grains between your hands. Drain off the cloudy water. Continue doing this until the water runs clear. Leave to drain or dry off the rice in a tea towel.
2 Into a large saucepan put ½ tbsp vegetable oil and heat to medium. Now add the rice and stir it around in the oil for 2 minutes, stirring all the time. Do not allow to burn.
3 Add the boiling water and salt, bring to a boil and continue a fast boil for 30 minutes or until the rice is tender.
4 When the rice is cooked, drain it into a sieve and rinse it with hot water.
5 Reheat the sauce and add the chopped coriander or parsley. Add to the rice on the plate. If you wish, serve with a side helping of vegetables.

Rabbit casserole
Serves 2

Rabbit is more easily digested than red meat and it contains little fat. Although it is rich in protein, it is best combined with vegetables because it is not a good source of vitamins or minerals.

Ingredients

1 small rabbit
3 shallots or 1 medium onion,
  finely chopped
1 tbsp olive oil
1 tsp paprika
salt and pepper to taste

150 ml (¼ pint) apple juice and
  150 ml (¼ pint) hot water
gluten-free flour for dusting the
  rabbit joints
3 carrots
broccoli florets or peas (as desired)

Method

1 Joint the rabbit (but leave out the ribs – they can always be used for stock).
2 Dip the joints in a mixture of flour, seasoned with salt, pepper and paprika.
3 Fry the shallots in the olive oil until soft.
4 Add the rabbit joints to the onions and cook on high heat until browned, turning frequently.
5 Transfer to casserole dish, add the apple juice and hot water and place in oven at 180°C (350°F, gas mark 4) for 30 minutes, then reduce the heat and cook gently for a further 45 minutes.
6 While the rabbit is cooking, steam the sliced carrots and broccoli or peas until tender.

Rice soup
Serves 3–4

Technically this is a soup but it makes a very substantial meal.

Although it takes a longer time than some of the other recipes to cook, you do not have to be in attendance every minute. There is plenty of opportunity to get off your feet and into a nice relaxed position.

Ingredients

¾ cup brown rice
4 cups vegetable or fish stock, or gluten-free bouillon in 4 cups hot water
1½ tbsp tamari soy sauce
2 tsp mirin (a Japanese sweet rice wine made especially for cooking); if this is not easily available then use date syrup
2 spring onions, finely chopped

2 tsp sherry or sweet white wine (optional)
200 g (7 oz) chicken or prawns, cooked and chopped
2 eggs, lightly beaten
1 tsp ginger juice (3.75 cm (1½ inches) root ginger, peeled and grated and then squeezed will give you 1 tsp juice)

Method

1 Wash the rice until the water runs clear.
2 Combine the rice and stock in a large saucepan and bring to the boil. Cover, reduce the heat and simmer for 50 minutes. Check that the rice does not dry out; keep the liquid topped up.
3 Add the tamari soy sauce, the mirin and sherry or white wine, if using, and stir.
4 Add the chicken or prawns.
5 Remove from the heat. Just before serving stir in the egg and ginger juice and cook for 1 minute or until the egg just starts to set. Serve in soup bowls and sprinkle on the spring onion.

Lentil dhal with cauliflower
Serves 4

Pulses and beans need to be picked over for small stones and pieces of grit. The easiest way to do this is to spread a single layer on a large dinner plate and pick out any pieces before transferring the lentils to a sieve. You may have to do this two or three times depending on how many you are using. When they have been picked over, wash them through in the sieve. This gets rid of any surface dust or dirt. Red lentils do not need to be soaked like other pulses and beans. They boil down to a purée and will take up the flavours of added spices. No recipes that use dried pulses and beans other than lentils or split peas are included here because of the more lengthy preparation time needed for these other pulses and beans.

Ingredients

250 g (8 oz) red lentils
850 ml (1½ pints) water
1 tsp turmeric
2 tsp grated fresh ginger
2 tsp cumin seeds
1 tsp ground cumin
½ tsp ground black pepper
3 tbsp lemon juice

3 tbsp vegetable oil
¼ tsp chilli flakes, if desired
3 medium tomatoes, washed and
   quartered
7.5 cm (3 inches) sweet potato,
   washed, peeled and cubed
250 g (8 oz) cauliflower florets
olive oil, to drizzle

Method

1 Put the water in a large saucepan and set over a high heat. Bring to the boil and add the lentils and turmeric, and continue boiling until the lentils are soft, stirring occasionally.
2 Heat the oil, and fry the ginger, chilli flakes, cumin seeds and cumin powder for a few seconds.
3 Add the chopped sweet potato and cauliflower. Turn the vegetables with a spoon for 4 or 5 minutes until they become flecked with brown spots.
4 Add the tomato wedges, cover the pan and cook for 7–8 minutes, stirring every 2 minutes or so, until the vegetables are tender.
5 Add the vegetables to the dhal, which should by now be quite thick. Season with pepper and salt if required. Mix together all the ingredients gently but quickly.
6 Squeeze the lemon juice over the mixture and drizzle on some olive oil. Simmer until the grains have absorbed all the liquid, then serve.

Pak choi with tuna and sesame seeds
Serves 2

Ingredients

1 medium egg (white only),
   beaten
1 tbsp tamari soy sauce
2 tuna steaks, 2 cm (¾ inch) thick
2 tbsp sesame seeds
2 tbsp sesame oil or vegetable oil

1 garlic clove, finely chopped
1 shallot or 1 small onion, finely
   chopped
2 pak choi, cut in half lengthwise
juice of 1 lime

Method

1 Whisk the egg white and soy sauce together. Dip the tuna steaks in the mixture, one side only, then dip the steaks in the sesame seeds.
2 Heat 1 tbsp oil in heavy-based frying pan or wok. Cook the steaks, seed side first, for 3 minutes each side. Remove the tuna from the pan and keep warm.
3 Heat the remaining oil and fry the garlic and shallot until soft.
4 Add the pak choi and stir-fry for 2–3 minutes.
5 Pour over the lime juice and remove from the pan.
6 Serve the tuna steaks on top of the pak choi.

As an option you can use duck, chicken or turkey breasts instead of tuna steaks.

Light meals and snacks

Elsewhere in the book I talk about the value of eating little but often, perhaps having four to six light meals in a day. This places less strain on the digestive system and provides a steady supply of nutrition throughout the day, thereby limiting fatigue, increasing relaxation and ensuring that blood sugar levels are kept at a point where you can meet any physical demands made on you. At first on this regime I found it difficult to assess what to eat and how much. However, within a few days I had adjusted to the change and found that I had more energy and that my body felt so much better. The recipes and quantities below have been arrived at as a result of experience over the years.

A number of the recipes rely on bread. If you have found that wheat or gluten are triggers for your pain, or you are otherwise sensitive to them, then consider using gluten-free bread, which is now easily obtainable from most of the larger supermarkets (though as yet it is rather expensive). It can be bought as white bread, brown bread and bread to which has been added small seeds or grains. All of them need to be 'refreshed' by either warming in the microwave or toasting. I prefer toasting because the bread seems to hold together better when toasted, and also because toast was what I missed most when I had to give up bread after finding that I was sensitive to wheat and gluten. The alternative is to bake your own bread, either from ready-made gluten-free bread mixes or from gluten-free flours. With experience I have found that I prefer the reliability and texture of the bread mix made by Orgran. There are quite a number of gluten-free bread mixes on the market now, and which one you choose is very much a matter of taste. You can add your own small seeds and herbs if you wish.

Sandwich fillings, spreads, toppings and salad accompaniments

Tuna mayonnaise with tamari
Serves 2

Ingredients

1 130 g (4.5 oz) tin flaked tuna
dash tamari soy sauce
2 dessertspoons good-quality dairy-free mayonnaise

Method

1   Mix the tuna with the tamari, then add the mayonnaise.
2   Spoon on top of toast, baked potatoes, or serve with a small salad of chopped peppers and mixed green leaves.

Yoghurt with peppers and watercress
Serves 2

Dairy-free yoghurt is used in this recipe because it is more easily digested than milk-based yoghurt. If dairy-based products are used at all, they should be used in small quantities only, particularly if you are over-weight or have a high cholesterol level. Soya yoghurt is calming to the digestion and contains natural bacteria, which are vital to good digestion. Watercress is rich in vitamins and minerals, and it is helpful to anyone who has water retention and inflammation because it can act as a diuretic. Peppers, besides being rich in vitamins A and C and anti-oxidants, are good for the circulation.

Ingredients

4 tablespoons plain dairy-free yoghurt
bunch watercress, chopped
¼ red pepper, finely sliced and chopped
¼ green pepper, finely sliced and chopped
1 spring onion, chopped

Method

1   Mix all the dry ingredients gently into the yoghurt.
2   Season to taste (you can use ¼ tsp ground ginger as part of the seasoning).
3   Chill for 5 minutes and serve.

Tapenade

Ingredients

100 g (3½ oz) small green, stone-free olives

1 tbsp finely chopped herbs (tarragon, parsley, basil, oregano and dill can all be used, separately or in combination)

1 tbsp olive oil

juice of half a lemon

1 garlic clove, crushed

Method

Blend the olive oil, lemon juice and garlic in a food processor, together with the herbs. Add the olives to the mixture and continue to blend. Season to taste.

Use it on toast or in sandwiches (it goes well with egg sandwiches).

Guacamole

Ingredients

2 avocados

1 tsp grated onion

1 tsp lemon juice

2 tsp extra-virgin olive oil

pinch cayenne pepper or chilli powder

seasoning as required

Method

Peel and mash the avocados well. Blend in all the other ingredients and beat thoroughly.

Smokie pâté

Those of you who have read *Coping Successfully with Pain* will know that Eve and I lived for a number of years in the fishing quarter of Arbroath on the east coast of Scotland. We were surrounded by smoke houses producing the delicacy for which Arbroath is world renowned – the smokie! The smokie is a haddock that has been cured by hanging over wood smoke for a number of hours. The outer skin is a deep bronze colour and the flesh is pure white. It is delicious hot or cold. For the pâté we use it cold. If you cannot find an Arbroath smokie then you can substitute any naturally cured fish. Avoid any that have been artificially coloured with BFK ('brown for kippers' or E154) or that have had 'oak chemical flavourings' added. No seasoning is required – all the flavour comes from the fish.

Ingredients

flesh of 1 Arbroath smokie, roughly chopped or flaked
good-quality dairy-free mayonnaise

Method

Mix all ingredients together and serve on fingers of toast, or with a salad.

Other toppings

Another useful topping is nut butter – peanut, almond or hazelnut – which you can buy from your health-food shop. Many of the cheaper brands may contain a lot of salt so check the labels.

Crudités and dips

Crudités and dips are useful for snacking at any time and are much better for you than biscuits.

For crudités you can slice carrots, celery, courgettes, cucumber, spring onions or apple into 5 cm (2 inch) sticks.

For the dip, you can buy many varieties of houmous from most supermarkets and this makes a very nice dip. Just check on the label that there are no suspect additives.

Another basis for a good dip is plain soya yoghurt mixed with finely chopped chives, or cucumber and a little paprika; or you can use a blender to make your own using a little olive oil and lemon juice and adding chopped basil, coriander or parsley. There are many possible combinations, and it is well worthwhile trying out your own ideas.

Smoothies, juices and other drinks

Smoothies are a very good stand-by when you are trying to have four or more small meals a day and are trying to get in your five or more portions of fruit and vegetables. Smoothies are full of vitamins and do not take long to make if you have a blender. They use the whole fruit or vegetable rather than just the juice, so you get the fibre as well.

The recipe below uses melon, apple and ginger. Alternatives are nectarine and melon, or apple and pear with cinnamon instead of ginger. There is a non-alcoholic ginger drink available in health-food shops (advertised as having the kick of two very angry mules!), which is good by itself but can be added to fruit drinks instead of root or ground ginger.

Mango and apple is another alternative (you can buy unsweetened mango purée in some supermarkets; it is good mixed with soya milk in equal proportions). Blackberries or blackcurrants and apple make a juice that is very rich in vitamin C.

I also like mixed fruit and vegetable drinks, and I often use carrot with apple juice. If you can take citrus fruits, try carrot and orange. Carrot, celery and ginger also go well together. Apart from a high vitamin and mineral content, these drinks are excellent for clearing toxicity from the body. I often start the day with a vegetable juice or have a smoothie that is a combination of fruit and soya milk mid-morning or mid-afternoon. I count this as a light meal.

Do not worry if you do not have a blender. There are many different ready-made varieties on sale in supermarkets, although some contain citrus fruits and they can also be high in sugar, so your choice of flavours might be limited.

Melon, apple and ginger smoothie
Serves 2

I have tried various melon types but my preference is for the water-melon. However, you may like a sweeter drink, in which case I suggest galia, cantaloupe or honeydew melons. Melon is good for smoothies because it is a juicy fruit and therefore goes a long way.

Ingredients
half a large melon or a whole small melon
1 large eating apple
2.5 cm (1 inch) ginger, grated, or, ½ tsp ground ginger if fresh ginger is not available

Method
Cut and peel the fruit. Remove any seeds, cores and blemishes and cut into small chunks according to the type of equipment you are using for blending. Put all the ingredients together and blend for 30 seconds.

Desserts

When you are trying to do without cane sugar or to cut down on your calories, the first thing to go is usually the dessert! However, just now and then for a treat we can indulge ourselves. Here are just a few ideas for you to try.

Fruit salads

What about a fresh fruit salad, using your own favourites from apples, pears, cherries, grapes, pineapples, peaches, nectarines, black or red currants? Avoid citrus fruits and any other fruits that may be a trigger for your pain.

For a change, try stewed dried fruits such as unsulphured apricots, prunes, pears or apple rings. Wash dried fruit thoroughly and stone it if necessary. Put the fruit in a saucepan and pour over enough boiling water to cover. Bring to the boil then immediately lower the heat to a simmer. Cover with a lid and simmer gently until the fruit is just cooked. Do not overcook or you will end up with a mushy purée. Allow the fruit to cool and serve it topped with some non-dairy 'cream' or gluten-free ice-cream. (There is one on the market called Swedish Glace, which I like very much. It is dairy- and gluten-free.) For a change try sprinkling with finely chopped nuts or grated good-quality dark chocolate.

You have to be careful when eating dried fruit as it has double the sugars of fresh fruit.

Pancakes

These pancakes can also be used in savoury dishes.

Ingredients

275 ml (½ pint) soya milk
1 egg
pinch salt
1 tsp vegetable or olive oil

1 tbsp rice flour
1 tbsp millet flour or millet flakes
1 tbsp buckwheat flour (this is not related to wheat)

Method

You can make the batter very quickly by putting the milk, egg, salt and oil in a liquidizer and blending for 15–30 seconds. Then add the flours and blend for a further 30 seconds until the batter is smooth. If possible, let the batter stand for a while before you cook the pancakes.

Do not worry if you do not have a liquidizer – you can use the old-fashioned method: put the flours and salt into a bowl, beat together the egg, soya milk and oil, and pour this mixture gradually into the flours and salt, stirring all the time until smooth.

To cook, grease a frying pan or griddle with a little oil and when hot add 2 tablespoons (I find I get on better with a small ladle) of batter to the pan, quickly tipping the pan so that the batter spreads out evenly into a circle. Cook for 2–3 minutes over a medium heat, then turn the pancake over and cook for a further minute or two. Turn out on to a lightly oiled plate and keep warm in a moderately hot oven or under a low grill until you are ready to fill the pancakes. If you want to reheat them later then turn them on to a cool surface.

You can fill these pancakes with a sweet or savoury mix. Sweet ideas include fruit spread and warm cherries, served with dairy- and gluten-free ice-cream, non-dairy 'cream' or a small amount of apple or pear concentrate mixed in half a cup of hot water.

For a savoury pancake you can use tapenade, houmous, guacamole, mixed stir-fried vegetables, hot chopped tomatoes or, for a more sub-stantial dish, thinly sliced spring onions with shredded carrot and lettuce and dairy-free mayonnaise to which cubes of chicken have been added. One of my favourites is smoked salmon and mayonnaise. The choices are endless.

Prune and almond tart

Ingredients for the pastry base

30 g (1 oz) ground almonds	2 tbsp water
60 g (2 oz) rice flour	1 tbsp sunflower oil
¼ tsp cinnamon	2 tbsp tahini
⅛ tsp ground cloves	

Ingredients for the filling

60 g (2 oz) dried dates	2 tbsp gram flour (chickpea flour)
60 ml (2 fl oz) water	½ tsp almond essence
60 g (2 oz) soya spread	125 g (4 oz) pitted, ready-to-eat
125 g (4 oz) ground almonds	prunes
2 eggs	15 g (½ oz) flaked almonds

Method for the pastry

1 Place all the ingredients in a food processor and mix until the mixture forms crumbs. If you do not have a food processor, mix all the dry ingredients together, then the wet ingredients, then combine them with a fork.
2 Press the crumb mixture into the base of a greased 22 cm (9 inch) flan dish.
3 Bake the pastry in a pre-heated oven at 200°C (400°F, gas mark 6) for 15 minutes or until lightly browned.

Method for the filling

1 Finely dice the dates and simmer in the water until just soft.
2 Add the soya spread and allow it to soften, then add the ground almonds.
3 Beat the eggs and add to the mixture along with the gram flour and almond essence. Beat well or process until smooth.
4 Place the prunes on the pastry base (cut them in half if too large).
5 Place the almond mixture on top and smooth the surface.
6 Sprinkle with the flaked almonds and bake in a pre-heated 190°C (375°F, gas mark 5) oven for 20–25 minutes or until golden brown and firm to touch. Serve warm or cold with dairy-free ice-cream or soya 'cream'.

The tart is suitable for freezing.

Celebration fruit cake

This cake makes up for possibly feeling that you are left out at Christmas! It is a moist fruit cake that can be frozen in slices for later use.

Ingredients

175 g (6 oz) dried dates	60 g (2 oz) gluten-free cornflour
150 ml (5 fl oz) water	60 g (2 oz) soya flour
125 ml (4 fl oz) sunflower oil	2 tsp gluten-free baking powder
30 g (1 oz) ground almonds	60 g (2 oz) walnuts
1 tsp mixed spice	225 g (8 oz) raisins
juice of 1 orange	125 g (4 oz) carrot, grated
zest of 1 orange	1 apple, grated
60 g (2 oz) rice flour	

Method

1 Cut the dates into small pieces and place in a pan with the water. Simmer over a low heat for 10 minutes until the dates are soft. Allow to cool.
2 Place the dates, oil, ground almonds, mixed spice, eggs, orange juice and zest, the flours and the baking powder in a food processor and mix, or beat in a bowl until well blended.
3 Add the walnuts, raisins, grated carrot and grated apple, and stir in by hand.
4 Put the mixture into a pre-greased, lined 15–20 cm (6–8 inch) cake tin and bake in a pre-heated oven at 170°C (325°F, gas mark 3) for 30 minutes, then lower the temperature to 140°C (275°F, gas mark 1) and bake for another 45 minutes.
5 Allow the cake to cool in the tin for 10 minutes. Turn out on to a wire tray and remove the lining paper.

This cake will keep for 4 days, but if you wish cut it into slices and freeze them separately.

Hot beverages

Coffee and tea

Coffee and black tea are not usually recommended for chronic pain sufferers as they are potential triggers. Black tea has been fermented before drying and is therefore high in tannins, which makes it very acidic and so it can upset the digestive system. Traditionally in the UK people drink a lot of tea, and this is the danger. Perhaps one or two cups a day is acceptable but any more and the sensitivity of your system is increased. Like coffee, tea is also rich in caffeine, which can stimulate an already sensitive nervous system. If I drink coffee I have an immediate pain reaction, and for several hours my skin feels as though it is being crawled over by a multitude of spiders!

For the sake of your pain and your digestive system, try to wean yourself off these drinks and change to green tea or white tea, which are made from unfermented leaves. They lose none of the antioxidant qualities that are being claimed for the tea plant. Also try infusions of herbal teas, such as camomile tea, which has a calming effect, lemon and ginger tea or peppermint tea, both of which are good for the digestion. All of these drinks can be drunk without milk or sugar. Be careful of having too many of the more acidic herbal teas such as raspberry, strawberry, blackcurrant, fruits of the forest or any based on citrus fruits.

Drinking chocolate and malt drinks

All manufactured drinking chocolates and malt drinks contain milk and so are to be avoided.

Both milk and chocolate are well-known triggers for pain, particularly migraine and other headaches. If you can tolerate chocolate then you can make a drink using pure chocolate powder and soya or rice milk, but it can be very bitter.

Malt is usually made from wheat or barley and therefore is not to be recommended for anyone with a wheat or gluten problem.

12

Eating out

One of the first activities to be dropped when you first have chronic pain is eating out. It is difficult to sit comfortably for more than a few minutes, which means that you are unable to share fully in the experience of conversation and banter around the table. In my book *Coping Successfully with Pain*, I devote a lot of space to explaining how it is possible to regain the physical capability and desire to enjoy activities that have been lost, seemingly for ever. This chapter helps you to make the most of the experience of eating out by selecting foods that agree with you. I am assuming that you have reached a stage where you are able to think of venturing out. If not, you can regard this chapter as planning ahead in order to set goals for your future enjoyment when pain has been put in its rightful place as just a small part of your day-to-day experience.

If you are not troubled by allergies or food intolerance but you know that your pain is made worse if you eat certain things, then eating out should not be too much of a problem. However, you may still want to avoid dairy products, animal fats, red meats and wheat – known triggers for inflammation and pain.

Eating out can seem a daunting prospect if you are on a limited diet, and many people prefer not to take the risk: remember the woman I interviewed with coeliac problems who said that she avoided it as much as possible and only went out for a meal on rare occasions when she was invited by friends or for important family celebrations? If there was a choice on the menu she would choose what she thought would do least harm and risk the consequences of feeling ill and uncomfortable for a week or two. It need not be like that. Eve and I enjoy eating out, and it would take a lot for us to give up this pleasure. It means avoiding fast-food outlets, which presents no problems to us. The only way to find out if something is safe for you is to ask, and staff are usually only too pleased to check ingredients, especially if catering packs are being used. Remember, catering staff are very often untrained in providing for special diets. We find it safer to eat at a restaurant where a chef is preparing food from scratch as distinct from establishments that basically provide a full menu from ready-made catering packs. A chef will often come and talk to you about your needs and will often even suggest modifications to the menu or offer to prepare something for you. It helps to prepare yourself in advance by making a list of the foods that you can eat. Sometimes the modification needed only requires cooking in oil rather than butter or leaving out a sauce or dressing.

To make sure you get the best and safest possible service, try phoning ahead and stating your problem and asking if your needs can be met. Any good establishment will be able to prepare you something suitable if given sufficient notice.

A restaurant owner near our home always appreciated an advance call. He said it was common for people to turn up without prior notice of their problems and be completely inflexible about his menu.

I have had some amusing responses from waiting staff. Having asked for potatoes to be omitted from my order I have been asked, 'Will you have chips instead?' 'Sorry, I cannot eat bread because I am allergic to gluten' has been answered with, 'Would you like toast?' 'No, I won't have a sweet, thank you, I am allergic to milk' has yielded the answer, 'Then perhaps you would like a plain ice-cream.'

Generally I find it easier to eat out in Indian, Japanese or Asian restaurants.

Chinese restaurants

In Chinese establishments, of course, I have to specify that the food should contain no monosodium glutamate (MSG). MSG is used for thickening and flavouring but it tends to increase inflammation and can cause headaches for many people, whether they have a pain problem or not. It is easy for MSG to be left out because it is added during cooking, and not all Chinese restaurants and take-aways use it. Another thing to watch out for is soy sauce. There is only one variety that I know of that is wheat-free – tamari, of Japanese origin.

Be careful about ordering spring rolls or anything covered in pastry such as won tun. These were traditionally made with rice flour, on the premises, but now they are being bought in, in which case they are usually manufactured using wheat flour.

You may think that ordering a meal containing soya bean curd (tofu) would be safe, but even here you can find wheat has been added in factory manufacture. Always enquire whether there is wheat present in the tofu. Just remember too that many Chinese food outlets do not have a qualified cook on the staff. Most of the food is bought in ready-made and as a result you have to be more vigilant and be prepared to ask questions. If you are lucky enough to find a restaurant that suits you then stick with it.

The one thing you can be sure of is that Chinese restaurants will not be using dairy products. A high percentage of Chinese people, like the Japanese, are intolerant of milk.

Indian restaurants

My experience with restaurants and take-aways serving food from the Indian subcontinent is that they are more than willing to discuss all of the ingredients in a dish and to advise which contain milk, yoghurt, cream, wheat and ghee. Ghee is clarified butter but they also use a vegetable form of ghee, so if you see the word 'ghee' on the menu then ask which it is. More often than not nowadays the vegetable version is being used but it is important that you ask. I find that some Indian food has quite a high salt content so do not eat it too often. Bear in mind that take-away establishments tend to be generous in their portions – but you do not have to eat it all!

Japanese restaurants

In Japanese restaurants you have to be aware that the noodles are likely to be made from wheat. Of course it is possible to choose from a great variety of dishes that do not contain noodles. Japanese restaurants like to serve vegetables or fish coated in 'tempeh', a batter that is usually made from potato flour or rice flour – but it is always better to check. I have never had any problem with these items. The problems can come from condiments such as soy sauce (if not tamari) and, in particular, Japanese green mustard, which contains wheat and vinegar.

Thai restaurants

Like some Chinese establishments, Thai restaurants may also be buying in ready-made spring rolls, which contain wheat. Always ask. Thai restaurants do not seem to use monosodium glutamate in their cooking, but as with Chinese food, be sure the tofu does not contain wheat.

Of all the forms of Eastern cooking, I prefer Thai because the food is so delicately blended.

Omelettes

A word of caution! If you are sensitive to anything made with milk but can eat eggs, please note that omelettes generally now contain milk or butter (or both), whether you are eating out at home or abroad. I never eat an omelette in a restaurant unless I am able to discuss the ingredients with the chef to ensure that it is made without milk and butter. Some of the fast-food outlets use packet mixes, which are likely to contain dairy ingredients as well as other chemicals to which you might be sensitive.

Eating out abroad – and why not?

The whole purpose of this chapter is to encourage anyone who has pain or food sensitivities to live life to the full. Anyone with pain will have suffered many restrictions in their life involving work, holidays, friendships, sport and the enjoyment of many things that other people take for granted. Although you may have started getting back into more adventurous ways at home, you may still be a little afraid of going abroad. On several occasions I have received mail from readers of *Coping Successfully with Pain* who are full of enthusiasm as a result of having achieved enough confidence to venture abroad. One correspondent spoke of having the honeymoon she never expected. She had been married for three years, most of them in pain. Her husband planned a surprise visit to Paris, where they had originally planned to go on their honeymoon.

It is important to make plans and follow them through. Being able to make plans for the future is a normal part of life. Have you stopped making plans as a result of your pain? It is important to enjoy new experiences, sights, sounds and tastes and, perhaps more importantly, to experience warmer climates and probably notice the improvement in your condition. This involves a great deal of planning, not least financial, and perhaps making changes to your usual spending pattern. If, like me, you have retired, there is time to spend long periods away from home in the winter months. There are savings to be made on heating bills. The greatest bonus is in fitness. If I spend a winter in the UK I lose fitness, become less mobile, put on weight and experience more pain. When I take myself off to a warmer, sunnier climate, the weather is usually drier, which means that I spend more time outdoors and get more exercise by walking, cycling or swimming every day. When I am away my diet is based mainly on fresh vegetables and freshly caught seafood.

It is not just people who have dietary problems who have difficulty eating out abroad. If you spend your holiday on the Spanish Costas you will have seen many eating places advertising 'real English fish and chips', 'roast beef and Yorkshire pudding', 'Lancashire hotpot', 'cream teas', 'English ale' and 'real English tea', and some people will be tempted to go for something that they know rather than take a risk with 'foreign' food. It is not just the British who seek out the familiar. Whatever the nationality, people tend to seek out places that serve food that they recognize. Some will even go to a fast-food outlet where they can get burgers and chips or fish and chips. However, before you go to any foreign country it is as well to prepare yourself by purchasing a phrase book or dictionary in which you can at least look up the names of foods displayed on a menu.

Making preparations

If you have long-term pain, preparations for spending time away are much more important than they otherwise would be. No one wants to go on holiday and find that the experience is a terrible ordeal from start to finish. Planning is the key to enjoying a good holiday. Think about your destination. People with long-term pain, particularly with arthritis, do not usually take kindly to extremely high temperatures and high humidity. Think carefully about the season of the year and the temperatures that you are likely to experience. Is there easy walking? Is it hilly or rocky? This is something that I have to think about because I am not good on slopes or uneven ground and since I like to cycle when I am on holiday I look for a flat area, preferably with designated cycle paths.

The main problem with travel is finding a way in which you can have as much control as possible. Most forms of public transport have their limitations. Public transport takes away your control and puts you in the hands of other people. This means it is difficult to pace your day. You cannot always determine the length of time that you sit or stand, the times of eating and drinking, toilet visits, whether or not you get help with luggage. Two or three years ago we decided on a five-day trip to Paris, a place I had not visited for 25 years – before I had serious pain and mobility problems. The trip was a disappointment. The city seemed so much bigger! On the Metro, great flights of steps, long passageways and jostling crowds reduced me to exhaustion so that I was not able to make the visits to the places of interest that I had planned.

Travelling by air

Try to avoid long flights. They have many disadvantages for anyone with chronic pain. Unless you are rich and can afford to upgrade then you are likely to be in economy class and therefore to spend many hours in one position. My limit is a two-hour flight. Even then I have to make sure that the hours spent at the airport are as comfortable as possible and that wheelchair assistance is pre-booked. The other problem with flying is the food. Airline food is a problem to anyone with pain, and there are additional difficulties in making sure that you have enough water to drink during the flight. It is even more important to avoid alcohol when you are flying. Alcohol and flying are not the best companions even for fit people because of the likelihood of dehydration. The 'air-conditioning' may not in fact be putting out fresh air but recirculated air, and if you have a weak immune system you are more likely to catch infections.

Travelling by coach

If you are travelling by coach, think about the start time and get as much information as you can about travelling time between stops. Do you have to handle your own luggage? Take the precaution of carrying sufficient food for the journey because eating stops will probably be at motorway services where the menu is often limited and the food of the wrong sort for anyone with food sensitivities. If your destination is a hotel then inform your holiday provider in advance of your dietary needs and confirm that the hotel can meet them. If going on a self-catering holiday carry any essential food items that you may need and that you may not be able to buy locally.

In order to maintain maximum control over our journey, the meals en route and the pace of the day, Eve and I choose where possible to travel in our motor home. The only deadlines that we fix are for ferry crossings, because we prefer to drift from place to place and enjoy whatever the countryside offers. We avoid long spells at the wheel. We each spend only an hour driving at any time and we always make a stop after two hours for exercise, food and drink. As a general rule we do not travel for more than four hours in any one day. This ensures that we feel comfortable at the end of the day and are able to look forward to a pleasant evening meal. We often meet couples who tell us that the one with pain does no driving and the other one insists on virtually non-stop driving to get to their final destination, however far that may be. As someone with chronic pain, you can just think of what it must feel like at the end of such a journey.

Spain

People from northern Europe who go on holidays in different parts of the world often seek out cafés that provide familiar meals – sausages, chips, beef, lamb, pork chops and mashed and roast potatoes. If they are on a self-catering holiday then this is what they cook for themselves.

You will have heard of the much praised Mediterranean diet with its emphasis on vegetables, fruit, olives and olive oil, fish, seafood and a limited amount of meat and dairy produce; for me the Mediterranean countries are ideal places to visit. The fact that olive oil is used in cooking is a real bonus. If you are on a self-catering holiday, it is still possible at the weekly farmers' markets to find freshly picked vegetables grown organically by traditional methods. If you visit Spain you cannot fail to see row upon row of cured hams hanging up in specialist food shops and supermarkets. The best, and the most expensive, of these are Serrano and Iberico hams. They are cured without the help of any chemicals whatsoever and are derived from pigs fed only on acorns; as a result they contain little or no cholesterol. I avoid all other red meat and red meat products – these hams are the one exception because I find that I have no adverse reactions to them in small amounts.

It is well worthwhile experimenting with foods that are unfamiliar to you. When we do this we are often well rewarded by the experience. Salads are a speciality in Spain and most people start their meal with a salad. It is a common sight to see groups of young manual workers tucking in to a large salad at lunchtime as a prelude to their main course. You will be offered a choice of up to five or six different salads, some with meat, some with fish or seafood, some with cheese and some simple green salads. They are a far cry from the traditional British lettuce leaves, tomato and cucumber. When eating out in Spain I find the only real precautions that I have to take relate to avoiding anything in breadcrumbs, red meats and cheap offers of paella!

However, even in Spain, the fast-food outlets are being frequented more and more by young people, and in recent years there has been a marked increase in obesity and heart disease. It has now become a matter for national concern. I include this information to demonstrate that the Mediterranean diet is part of a way of life in which over-indulgence is not encouraged.

France

The French reputation for cuisine is well deserved at any level. It is possible to find a menu or a special dish to suit almost any dietary needs, and if what you need is not on the menu, the staff are only too willing to prepare you something special and, more often than not, you need not worry about the language. Sometimes I find it difficult to practise my French because many restaurant staff are pleased to show their knowledge of English. When travelling we tend to look out for the Géant supermarkets. They are well signposted in most large towns and at lunchtime the Casino self-service restaurant that forms part of the supermarket complex provides a selection of foods, beautifully presented. It is always possible to find something suitable and enjoyable to eat. The meals are very economical in price. Other supermarket chains provide the same sort of service at their larger stores. The hotel chain Logis de France provides a map showing the location of their eating establishments. Their trademark is a green and yellow sign showing one, two or three chimneys – the more chimneys, the more expensive the meals. Whether you go to a one-, two- or three-chimney establishment, you can be sure of enjoying local produce that is well cooked and presented at an economical price. Motorways also serve excellent meals and offer quite a different eating experience from any motorway services in the UK. However, do not be tempted to accept anything that is on offer rather than engage in conversation about your eating requirements.

Other things to consider when travelling in Europe

There is a great awareness of dietary problems on the Continent and you often find that the person serving you has a family member or a friend with a similar problem. There are one or two notes of caution. If you are in the north of France and you wish to have *moules frites* (mussels and chips), for example, you will probably find that butter is used in the recipe, whereas in the south oil is used. Therefore, when you order it is wise to check whether or not dairy produce is included. Similarly, butter may be used to glaze vegetables or to grill fish, and it does no harm to check this with the staff if butter causes you a problem.

When I eat in other parts of Europe – for example, Germany, Switzerland, the Netherlands, Belgium or Italy – I find that there is a lot more emphasis on dairy products and meat. In Germany in particular there is much more emphasis on red meat dishes – in large servings. My inclination here is always to seek out a Chinese restaurant or find somewhere that serves fish. In Switzerland the emphasis is more on cheese and cream and here again I search out Chinese or Thai restaurants, but having said that, near the lakes it is possible to enjoy some delicious fish dishes. As a general rule, if you are in a dairy-producing country then you will be offered more cheese, cream, yoghurt and red meat. You can get along by being aware of your trigger foods and avoiding rich sauces and food cooked in butter. The Netherlands is similarly dominated by dairy produce but fortunately there is a plentiful supply of fish and vegetables.

I have never found Italy an easy country in which to eat out because traditional Italian cooking is based on wheat, cheese, cream and tomatoes. On the few occasions that I have visited restaurants in Italy, I have tried to find fish or seafood dishes accompanied by roasted vegetables.

Cruising

Cruising holidays are becoming increasingly popular as a 'get-away-from-it-all' break, particularly for people who are less mobile. The real danger of going on a cruise is that you are tempted to over-indulge in red meat, rich dairy-based dishes and alcohol throughout the day and well into the night! It takes a lot of discipline when you are faced with five-course breakfasts, seven-course lunches and dinners, midnight buffets and bars and cafés that open all day for drinks and snacks. If you are at sea for any length of time you can be sorely tempted to indulge yourself out of boredom or for purely social reasons.

It is possible to go on a cruise with a pain problem and gain benefit from the experience but you must plan ahead and liaise with the cruise company's customer services department, letting them know precisely what your dietary needs are, well in advance of the start of the cruise. You will appreciate that your food will have to be taken on board before you leave port. The crew will not be able to drop off to pick up soya milk in the middle of the Atlantic. Eve and I went on a cruise some years ago to celebrate a wedding anniversary and were most impressed by the service we received. The head waiter was assigned to discuss the menu before every meal and to ensure that I was protected from accidentally ordering something unsuitable. I had to impose my own discipline on the frequency and quantity of the food I ate.

13

Conclusion

I want to stress that food alone is not sufficient to fight chronic pain but it can do much to ease the symptoms and promote healing. You will still need to pay attention to your lifestyle, and the way you think, emphasizing positive thoughts, setting yourself manageable goals, exercising, pacing yourself and following a relaxation programme. However, unless you take responsibility for making an individual assessment of your nutritional needs, everything else that you do will be undermined.

For example, Paul damaged his spine 10 years ago in a car accident. He developed arthritis and is on strong pain-killers and anti-inflammatory drugs because he is in constant pain. He also suffers from diabetes and now has a heart problem.

He seeks solace in eating. In spite of his problems he eats a large lunch, which includes steak and chips followed by an elaborate ice-cream dessert. Mid-morning will see him in a café eating a bacon sandwich before setting off to find a chip shop! Of course he is overweight. I asked him about this destructive behaviour, which is not helping his arthritis, diabetes or heart problems. He said that he knew that the drugs he was on were doing so much damage to his liver and kidneys that he could not look forward to a long life so while he was waiting he would eat what and when he fancied it. He had no idea that by making small changes to his diet and controlling his appetite, he could prevent further deterioration in his condition and even see improvements in his general health. He needed help to see there were far greater pleasures in life than eating to excess and that it was within his power to begin the healing process.

What can Paul do to get out of this downward spiral? He is plainly overwhelmed by the whole situation and can only see a limited future for himself and so has sought refuge in comfort eating, which has got out of control. He feels he is in a helpless situation and that he must accept the inevitable consequences. In fact, with a little help, Paul's situation could be turned around. He could be encouraged to tackle his problem one step at a time. If you were in Paul's position what steps would you take?

1 You could have a talk with your doctor to see if your medication can be adjusted. Might it be this that is contributing to the eating problem?

2 Establish regular meal times and stop eating in between meals (that includes ice-creams).

3 Explore with your doctor the possibility of being referred to a pain management course. In the meantime, find ways of learning relaxation techniques. There are many books and audio discs on the market, and Pain Association Scotland have their own CDs for sale at a modest price.

4 Experiment with small changes in your diet as you try to identify foods that might be responsible for triggering your pain. Start by limiting or even cutting out red meat, dairy products and anything made from wheat. Try this for two weeks and see how you feel and note any improvement to your pain.

5 Try to increase the amount of fruit and vegetables that you eat each day.

6 Drink plenty of liquids, water, herbal teas or diluted sugar-free fruit juices.

7 If you have got into bad habits and are regulating your day around food, try to change your pattern – for instance, take a walk mid-morning in an area where you will not be tempted by sights and smells of food outlets.

There are, however, factors that might make change difficult. You might be wondering how you can manage without fry-ups, red meat, sausages, alcohol, and maybe cheese, milk, sugary foods and drinks, tea and coffee – and perhaps even your favourite bread. All you have to do at this stage is try one or two changes then move on from there. Do not forget that I have had 15 years to make these changes – and with each change the results have been positive for my pain and general health.

It is appreciated that you may be in a position where you do not have any control over the food you eat. You may be dependent on a partner or another close relative to prepare your meals and feel that you are putting a burden on them if you ask them to change your diet and make 'special' meals just for you. Perhaps you are in a residential establishment and find it difficult to make your needs known to the staff. Think about passing on this book to the management with a view to arranging some adjustment in your diet. If anyone reading this book has any part to play in the provision of residents' meals, or meals-on-wheels, consider how far your organization really caters for the needs of people who have chronic pain conditions. I know that vegetarian meals are provided but these often depend heavily on cheese and other dairy products.

In *Coping Successfully with Pain*, I stressed the importance of setting targets and working towards goals as a means of functioning from day to day in order to regain control of your life and to keep pain in a less dominant place. As time has passed, I have learned just how important it is to set goals for almost every aspect of your life. This advice is important for everyone, but it is even more important to anyone who carries the burden of chronic pain. It is crucial for increasing mobility, achieving deep relaxation, making lifestyle changes and meeting challenges. This way, life becomes so much more interesting. Do not set out to achieve great things immediately but proceed by taking small steps. When you succeed in the first small steps you will gain in confidence to become more ambitious. If you falter, this is probably a sign that you have set yourself too difficult a challenge and you will need to readjust your goal. If walking is a problem for you, then setting yourself increasing challenges each day is important. As you gain confidence and are able to walk for a longer period each day, then think about setting yourself a more challenging goal and plan to achieve it by succeeding at a number of intermediate targets. As you achieve your goals, you will become more confident in every area of your life. Adopt the same attitude towards your food, your body's fuel. Set goals for eating more healthily, and reduce your pain.

Appendix

Useful phrases when eating out abroad are given below in various languages.

Spanish

I am allergic to all dairy products including milk, cheese, cream, butter and yoghurt. Can you please advise me what is safe for me to eat from your menu?

Soy alergico a toda clase de productos lacteos: leche, queso, nata, mantequilla y yogurt. ¿Por favor, informeme qué puedo tomar de su menu?

I am allergic to wheat flour and gluten. Can you please advise me what is safe to eat from your menu?

Soy alergico a la harina de trigo y al gluten. ¿Puede aconsejarme sobre lo que puedo comer de su menu?

It is dangerous for me to eat nuts!

Es peligroso para mi tomar nueces, avellanas, cacahuetes, etc!

I am unable to eat red meat.

Soy incapaz de tomar carnes rojas – buey, vaca, tenera, cerdo, cordero.

Can you suggest something from your menu that will not cause me any problems?

¿Tal vez me pueda sugerir algo del menu que no me cause problemas?

I am unable to eat eggs.

No puedo comer heuvos.

Please do not use soy sauce.

No usen salsa de soja, por favor.

Please do not use monosodium glutamate.

No usen glutamate monosodico, por favor.

Please leave off the sauce/gravy.

Por favor, no mi ponga salsa.

Would you please grill the fish with olive oil only, and do not dust the fish with flour.

Por favor, podria tomar el pescado a la plancha con un poco de aceite de oliva. No reboze el pescado con harina.

I would like a herbal tea.

Me gustaria tomar una infusion de hierbas.

French

I am allergic to all dairy products.

Je suis allergique à tous les produits laitiers.

Can you please advise me what it is safe to eat from your menu?

Pouviez-vous me signaller les plats les plus adaptés pour moi du menu?

I am allergic to wheat flour and gluten.

Je suis allergique à la farine de blé et au gluten, s'il vous plaît.

It is dangerous for me to eat nuts.

C'est dangereux pour moi manger des noix, des noisettes, des cacahouetes, etc.

I am unable to eat red meat: beef, pork, lamb.

Je ne peux pas manger du boeuf, du porc, de l'agneau.

I am allergic to eggs.

Je suis allergique aux oeufs.

I can eat chicken, duck, turkey and rabbit and fish.

Je peux manger du poulet, du canard, du dindon et du lapin et du poisson.

Would you please grill the fish with a little olive oil only. Do not dust the fish with flour.

S'il vous plaît, pouviez-vous griller le poisson avec un peu de l'huile d'olive seulement. Ne pas utiliser de la farine en aucun cas.

I can eat all shellfish.

Je peux manger tous les fruits de mer.

I can eat all vegetables.

Je peux manger tous les légumes verts.

I can eat eggs.

Je peux manger des oeufs.

Please do not use vinegar.
S'il vous plaît, n'employez pas du vinaigre.

Please do not use soy sauce or monosodium glutamate.
Ne faites pas usage de la sauce soja, ou monosodium glutamate, s'il vous plaît.

Please leave off the sauce/gravy.
Je vous prie d'enlever la sauce.

I would like a herbal tea.
Je voudrais prendre une infusion, s'il vous plaît.

German

I am allergic to all dairy products including milk, cheese, cream and butter.
Ich bin allergisch gegen Milch und daraus hergestelle Produkte (Käse, Sahne, Butter).

I am allergic to wheat flour and gluten.
Ich bin allergisch gegen Weizenmehl und Gluten.

Can you recommend dishes that don't contain these products?
Können Sie mir Speisen empfehlen, die diese Produkte nicht enthalten?

It is dangerous for me to eat nuts.
Es ist gefährlich für mich alle Arten von Nüsse zu essen.

I am unable to eat beef.
Ich darf kein Rindfleisch essen.

I am unable to eat pork.
Ich darf kein Schweinefleisch essen.

I am unable to eat lamb or mutton.
Ich darf kein Lamm- oder Hammelfleisch essen.

I am unable to eat eggs.
Ich darf keine Eier essen.

I can eat chicken, duck, turkey and rabbit.
Ich darf Huhn, Ente, Pute und Kaninchen essen.

I can eat all fish.
Ich darf alle Fische essen.

Could you please grill the fish with a little olive oil only.
Würden Sie bitte den Fisch unpaniert mit etwas Olivenol braten (oder grillen).

I can eat all shellfish (mussels).
Ich darf alle Arten von Schalentieren (Muscheln) essen.

I can eat all vegetables.
Ich darf alle Gemüsesorten essen.

I can eat eggs.
Ich darf Eier essen.

Please do not use vinegar.
Bitte verwenden Sie keinen Essig.

Please do not use soy sauce.
Bitte verwenden Sie keine Sojasosse.

Please do not use monosodium glutamate.
Bitte verwenden Sie kein Glutamat.

Please leave off the sauce/gravy.
Bitte keine Sosse.

I would like a herbal tea.
Ich möchte einen Krautertee.

Dutch

I am allergic to all dairy products.
Ik ben allergisch voor alle melkproducten.

I am allergic to wheat flour and gluten.
Ik ben allergisch voor tarwe bloem en gluten.

Can you please advise what is safe for me to eat.
Kunt u mij adviseren wat voor mij veilig is om te eten?

It is dangerous for me to eat nuts.
Het is voor mij gevaarlijk om noten te eten.

I am unable to eat beef, pork, lamb and eggs.
Ik mag geen rund-, varkens-, en lamsvlees eten en ook geen eieren, ik ben daar allergisch voor.

I can eat chicken, duck, turkey and rabbit.
Ik mag wel kip, eend, kalkoen en konijn eten.

I can eat all fish.
Alle soorten vis mag ik eten.

Would you please grill the fish with a little olive oil only.
Wilt u alstublieft de vis grillen met alleen wat olijfolie?

I can eat all shellfish.
Schelpdieren mag ik wel eten.

I can eat all vegetables.
Ik mag alle soorten groenten eten.

Please do not use vinegar, soy sauce, monosodium glutamate.
Wilt u alstublieft geen azijn, sojasaus of monosodium glutamate gebruiken.

Please leave off the sauce/gravy.
Wilt u alstublieft de saus of de jus weglaten.

I would like a herbal tea.
Ik wil graag kruidenthee.

Italian

I am allergic to all dairy products including milk, cheese, cream and butter.
Sono allergico a tutti i prodotti caseari incluso il latte, formaggio, panna e burro.

I am unable to eat red meat.
Non posso mangiare carne rossa.

I am allergic to wheat and gluten.

Sono allergico a tutte le farine ed al glutine.

Would you please grill or fry the fish with some oil but do not dust it with flour.

Potrebbe, per favore, grigliare o friggere il pesce con dell'olio ma non usi nessun genere di farina.

I am allergic to egg.

Sono allergico alle uova.

I am allergic to nuts.

Sono allergico alle noci.

Useful addresses and further reading

Useful adresses

Allergy UK
3 White Oak Square
London Road
Swanley
Kent BR8 7AG
Tel.: 01322 619898
Website: www.allergyuk.org

Arthritis Care
18 Stephenson Way
London NW1 2HD
Tel.: 020 7380 6500
Information Line (for information pack and general details): 0845 600 6868
Helpline: 0808 800 4050 (10 a.m. to 4 p.m. weekdays)
Helpline via email: helplines@arthritiscare.org.uk
Website: www.arthritiscare.org.uk

Also provides community-based management courses.

BackCare
The Old Office Block
16 Elmtree Road
Teddington
Middlesex TW11 8ST
Tel.: 020 8977 5474
Helpline: 0845 130 2704
Website: www.backcare.org.uk

Biotech Health and Nutrition Centre
Worcester House
4 Dragon Street
Petersfield
Hants GU31 4JD
Tel.: 01730 233414
Website: www.nutrivital.co.uk

This organization conducts tests on all aspects of nutrition and environmental illness, and has fully trained practitioners throughout the country.

British Dietetics Association
Fifth Floor, Charles House
148–149 Great Charles Street
Birmingham B3 3HT
Tel.: 0121 200 8080
Website: www.bda.uk.com
Email: info@bda.uk.com

Institute for Complementary Medicine
Unit 25, Tavern Quay Business Centre
Sweden Gate
London SE16 7TX
Tel.: 020 7231 5855
Website: www.i-c-m.org.uk

Provides information on all complementary and professionally qualified
practitioners.

Institute for Optimum Nutrition (ION)
Avalon House
72 Lower Mortlake Road
Richmond
Surrey TW9 2JY
Tel.: 020 8614 7800
Website: www.ion.ac.uk
Email: reception@ion.ac.uk

Pain Association Scotland
Cramond House
Cramond Glebe Road
Kirk Cramond
Edinburgh EH4 6NS
Tel.: 0800 783 6059 (freephone helpline 9.30 a.m. to 4.30 p.m., Monday to
Friday, for people with chronic pain, including cancer pain)
Website: www.painassociation.com
Email: info@painassociation.com

This association provides courses throughout Scotland in the self-
management of chronic pain. They are the sole suppliers of relaxation
CDs recorded by the author.

Pain Concern
PO Box 13256
Haddington
Lothian EH41 4YD
Tel.: 01620 822572 (9 a.m. to 5 p.m., Monday to Friday. On Friday evening
from 6.30 to 7.30 the number provides a Listening Ear helpline for people
to talk to others in pain.)
Website: www.painconcern.org.uk
Email: info@painconcern.org.uk

This group is run by people who are themselves coping with chronic pain.

Further reading

Barnard, Dr N., *Foods That Fight Pain*. Bantam Books, London, 1999. The
book includes menus and recipes by Jennifer Raymond.
Brown, S., *Vegetarian Kitchen*. BBC, London, 1984 (new edn 1995).
Clucas, H. and Lindsay, A., *The Real Food of China*. William Heinemann,
Australia, 1988.
Cousins, B., *Vegetarian Cooking Without*. Thorsons, London, 2000.
Dasa, A., *The Hare Krishna Book of Vegetarian Cooking*. The Bhaktivedanta
Book Trust, Alachua, FL, 1984 (new edn 1990).
Gloaguen, Dr D., *Fatigue Chronique & Fibromyalgie*. Alpén Editions,
Monaco, 2007.
Holford, P., *The Optimum Nutrition Bible*. Piatkus, London, 1998 (updated
2004 under the title *The New Optimum Nutrition Bible*).
Lawrence, F., *Not On the Label*. Penguin, London, 2004.
Lawson, J., *A Little Taste of Japan*. Murdoch Books, Sydney, Australia, 2000.
Petit, H., *Le Mal de Dos, C'est Fini*. Alpén Editions, Monaco, 2005.
Quéquet, Dr C., *Vaincre L'Allergie*. Alpén Editions, Monaco, 2005.
Tétau, Dr M., *Rhumatismes: Votre Ordonnance Naturelle*. Alpén Editions,
Monaco, 2006.
Weil, Dr A., *Eating Well for Optimum Health*. Time Warner Paperbacks, New
York, 2001.
Wells, Dr C. and Nown, G., *The Pain Relief Handbook*. Vermilion, London,
1996.
Zukin, Jane, *Dairy-Free Cookbook*. Prima Publishing, Roseville, CA, (second
revd edn 1998).

Index